Mobile Point-of-Care Monitors and Diagnostic Device Design

Devices, Circuits, and Systems

Series Editor
Krzysztof Iniewski
CMOS Emerging Technologies Research Inc.,
Vancouver, British Columbia, Canada

PUBLISHED TITLES:

Atomic Nanoscale Technology in the Nuclear Industry
Taeho Woo

Biological and Medical Sensor Technologies
Krzysztof Iniewski

Building Sensor Networks: From Design to Applications
Ioanis Nikolaidis and Krzysztof Iniewski

Circuits at the Nanoscale: Communications, Imaging, and Sensing
Krzysztof Iniewski

Electrical Solitons: Theory, Design, and Applications
David Ricketts and Donhee Ham

Electronics for Radiation Detection
Krzysztof Iniewski

Embedded and Networking Systems: Design, Software, and Implementation
Gul N. Khan and Krzysztof Iniewski

Energy Harvesting with Functional Materials and Microsystems
Madhu Bhaskaran, Sharath Sriram, and Krzysztof Iniewski

Graphene, Carbon Nanotubes, and Nanostuctures: Techniques and Applications
James E. Morris and Krzysztof Iniewski

High-Speed Devices and Circuits with THz Applications
Jung Han Choi and Krzysztof Iniewski

High-Speed Photonics Interconnects
Lukas Chrostowski and Krzysztof Iniewski

Integrated Microsystems: Electronics, Photonics, and Biotechnology
Krzysztof Iniewski

Integrated Power Devices and TCAD Simulation
Yue Fu, Zhanming Li, Wai Tung Ng, and Johnny K.O. Sin

Internet Networks: Wired, Wireless, and Optical Technologies
Krzysztof Iniewski

Low Power Emerging Wireless Technologies
Reza Mahmoudi and Krzysztof Iniewski

PUBLISHED TITLES:

Medical Imaging: Technology and Applications
Troy Farncombe and Krzysztof Iniewski

MEMS: Fundamental Technology and Applications
Vikas Choudhary and Krzysztof Iniewski

Microfluidics and Nanotechnology: Biosensing to the Single Molecule Limit
Eric Lagally and Krzysztof Iniewski

MIMO Power Line Communications: Narrow and Broadband Standards, EMC, and Advanced Processing
Lars Torsten Berger, Andreas Schwager, Pascal Pagani, and Daniel Schneider

Mobile Point-of-Care Monitors and Diagnostic Device Design
Walter Karlen and Krzysztof Iniewski

Nano-Semiconductors: Devices and Technology
Krzysztof Iniewski

Nanoelectronic Device Applications Handbook
James E. Morris and Krzysztof Iniewski

Nanopatterning and Nanoscale Devices for Biological Applications
Krzysztof Iniewski and Seila Šelimović

Nanoplasmonics: Advanced Device Applications
James W. M. Chon and Krzysztof Iniewski

Nanoscale Semiconductor Memories: Technology and Applications
Santosh K. Kurinec and Krzysztof Iniewski

Novel Advances in Microsystems Technologies and Their Applications
Laurent A. Francis and Krzysztof Iniewski

Optical, Acoustic, Magnetic, and Mechanical Sensor Technologies
Krzysztof Iniewski

Radiation Effects in Semiconductors
Krzysztof Iniewski

Semiconductor Radiation Detection Systems
Krzysztof Iniewski

Smart Grids: Clouds, Communications, Open Source, and Automation
David Bakken and Krzysztof Iniewski

Smart Sensors for Industrial Applications
Krzysztof Iniewski

Technologies for Smart Sensors and Sensor Fusion
Kevin Yallup and Krzysztof Iniewski

Telecommunication Networks
Eugenio Iannone

PUBLISHED TITLES:

Testing for Small-Delay Defects in Nanoscale CMOS Integrated Circuits
Sandeep K. Goel and Krishnendu Chakrabarty

Wireless Technologies: Circuits, Systems, and Devices
Krzysztof Iniewski

FORTHCOMING TITLES:

3D Circuit and System Design: Multicore Architecture, Thermal Management, and Reliability
Rohit Sharma and Krzysztof Iniewski

Circuits and Systems for Security and Privacy
Farhana Sheikh and Leonel Sousa

CMOS: Front-End Electronics for Radiation Sensors
Angelo Rivetti

Gallium Nitride (GaN): Physics, Devices, and Technology
Farid Medjdoub and Krzysztof Iniewski

High Frequency Communication and Sensing: Traveling-Wave Techniques
Ahmet Tekin and Ahmed Emira

Labs-on-Chip: Physics, Design and Technology
Eugenio Iannone

Laser-Based Optical Detection of Explosives
Paul M. Pellegrino, Ellen L. Holthoff, and Mikella E. Farrell

Metallic Spintronic Devices
Xiaobin Wang

Nanoelectronics: Devices, Circuits, and Systems
Nikos Konofaos

Nanomaterials: A Guide to Fabrication and Applications
Gordon Harling, Krzysztof Iniewski, and Sivashankar Krishnamoorthy

Optical Fiber Sensors and Applications
Ginu Rajan and Krzysztof Iniewski

Organic Solar Cells: Materials, Devices, Interfaces, and Modeling
Qiquan Qiao and Krzysztof Iniewski

Power Management Integrated Circuits and Technologies
Mona M. Hella and Patrick Mercier

Radio Frequency Integrated Circuit Design
Sebastian Magierowski

Semiconductor Device Technology: Silicon and Materials
Tomasz Brozek and Krzysztof Iniewski

FORTHCOMING TITLES:

Soft Errors: From Particles to Circuits
Jean-Luc Autran and Daniela Munteanu

VLSI: Circuits for Emerging Applications
Tomasz Wojcicki and Krzysztof Iniewski

Wireless Transceiver Circuits: System Perspectives and Design Aspects
Woogeun Rhee and Krzysztof Iniewski

Mobile Point-of-Care Monitors and Diagnostic Device Design

EDITED BY

Walter Karlen

University of British Columbia, Vancouver, British Columbia, Canada

Krzysztof Iniewski MANAGING EDITOR

CMOS Emerging Technologies Research Inc., Vancouver, British Columbia, Canada

CRC Press
Taylor & Francis Group
Boca Raton London New York

CRC Press is an imprint of the
Taylor & Francis Group, an **informa** business

CRC Press
Taylor & Francis Group
6000 Broken Sound Parkway NW, Suite 300
Boca Raton, FL 33487-2742

ISBN 13: 978-1-4665-8929-2 (hbk)

Visit the Taylor & Francis Web site at
http://www.taylorandfrancis.com

and the CRC Press Web site at
http://www.crcpress.com

Contents

Preface

Shortages of skilled medical personnel and increasing costs present a challenge to health care systems around the world. Particularly in remote and resource poor areas, long travel distances to hospitals and lengthy laboratory results turnaround times delay diagnosis and treatment of severe infectious and noninfectious diseases. Ubiquitous mobile systems that allow for monitoring of vital signs, diagnosis, and treatment of diseases at the point-of-care facility can provide an effective means of addressing these global challenges. In parallel, the omnipresence and connectivity of mobile phones and consumer electronics allows lay users to collect, access, and manage personal health information everywhere. Mobile health (mHealth) and personal health (pHealth) are emerging research topics that bring electronic health (eHealth) and point-of-care monitoring to a new dimension. Important clinical tests can be performed on a mobile device conveniently outside the hospital at home, and test results are available immediately. These are exciting new opportunities for researchers, engineers, software developers, medical personnel, health care providers, and regulatory bodies.

Point-of-care medical diagnostics also poses new challenges. Sensor design for mobile devices requires particular attention, as low power consumption, compactness, and robustness are desired, while maintaining accuracy and sensitivity are crucial. Signal processing and classification is being challenged by increased levels of noise and artifacts as devices are being used in everyday settings outside the controlled hospital and laboratory environments. As patients with no advanced medical training are being empowered with sensors and devices to monitor their own health, user interfaces, measurement procedures, and work flows have to be simplified to reduce information overload. This calls for extended usability testing, interactive and embedded device training, and research on implementation and deployment. Health care providers also need to be informed about screening results and the quality of the assessments, leveraging the networking capabilities of devices while maintaining a high level of data security and confidentiality. The contributors to this book have all made significant contributions to important fields in point-of-care system development and/or deployment and we are proud to present their research here.

We cover two main research topics of particular interest to point-of-care device developers and implementers. In Part 1, we provide an overview of recent advances in sensing technologies for mobile point-of-care instruments. Innovations and new design trends for sensors and systems are illustrated and the authors provide new insights into state-of-the art technology for portable diagnostics. In the first three chapters, we discuss how to design lab-on-chip devices and vital-sign monitors, and we show how to cost effectively connect them to consumer devices. These technologies have high application potential in low-resource settings where current screening approaches are not available. Chapters 4 and 5 discuss fundamental research on sensor technology that demonstrates a great potential for implementation in point-of-care testing.

In Part 2, we provide new insights into research and methodologies for designing personal diagnostic and point-of-care devices and bringing them to market. Essential approaches for successful biomedical information processing are highlighted, with two chapters describing successful approaches for obtaining regulatory approval and testing usability of point-of-care devices. These chapters focus not only on established North American markets, but on other strategies for emerging markets as well.

This book offers a valuable resource to biomedical engineers, researchers, and health professionals who want to stay updated with recent advances in point-of-care device developments.

Editors

Walter Karlen, Ph.D., earned a M.Sc. degree in micro-engineering (2005) and a Ph.D. in computer communication and information sciences (2009) from École Polytechnique Fédérale de Lausanne (EPFL), Switzerland. He currently holds an advanced research fellowship from the Swiss National Science Foundation and is co-hosted by the Electrical and Computer Engineering in Medicine research group (ecem.ece.ubc.ca) at the Child and Family Research Institute and the Department of Electrical and Computer Engineering of the University of British Columbia (UBC) in Vancouver, Canada and by the Biomedical Engineering Research Group at the Department of Mechanical and Mechatronic Engineering at the University of Stellenbosch, South Africa. Dr. Karlen is an awardee of the Rising Stars in Global Health program of Grand Challenges Canada. In 2013, he was awarded the Killam Postdoctoral Fellow Research Prize by UBC.

Dr. Karlen's objective is to enable the diagnosis, monitoring, and treatment of major global health burdens by developing personalized methods, devices, and efficient systems that can be used at the point of care. His current projects include the implementation of biomedical sensors on mobile phones for global health applications. His research focuses on the technical aspects of mobile health and point-of-care devices such as real-time biomedical signal processing, mobile computing, sensors and systems design, and quality control. He also focuses on the improvement of clinical decision support with the design of adaptive systems, smart alarms, and optimized user-machine interaction. One of his successful projects, the Phone Oximeter (www.phoneoximeter.org), allows for the monitoring of vital signs with a mobile phone in rural areas away from medical centers. Within current pilot projects, the Phone Oximeter monitors sick children and mothers and provides diagnostic support to health workers in Uganda, South Africa, India, and Bangladesh. In Vancouver, the Phone Oximeter has been clinically tested at British Columbia Children's Hospital to monitor children with respiratory sleep problems. Dr. Karlen can be reached at www.karliwalti.ch and walter.karlen@ieee.org.

Krzysztof (Kris) Iniewski, Ph.D., manages R&D at Redlen Technologies, Inc., a startup company in Vancouver, Canada. Redlen's revolutionary production process for advanced semiconductor materials enables a new generation of more accurate, all-digital, radiation-based imaging solutions. Kris is also president of CMOS Emerging Technologies Research, Inc. (www.cmosetr.com), an organization of high-tech events covering communications, microsystems, optoelectronics, and sensors. Dr. Iniewski has held numerous faculty and management positions at University of Toronto, University of Alberta, Simon Fraser University (SFU), and PMC-Sierra, Inc. He has published over 100 research papers in international journals and conferences. He holds 18 international patents granted in the United States, Canada, France, Germany, and Japan. He is a frequent invited speaker and has consulted for multiple organizations internationally. He has written and edited several books for

CRC Press, Cambridge University Press, IEEE Press, Wiley, McGraw Hill, Artech House, and Springer. His personal goal is to contribute to healthy living and sustainability through innovative engineering solutions. In his leisure time Kris can be found hiking, sailing, skiing, or biking in beautiful British Columbia. He can be reached at kris.iniewski@gmail.com.

Contributors

Alfred Andama
College of Health Sciences
Makerere University
Kampala, Uganda

Grace Bartoo
Decus Biomedical, LLC
Berkeley, California

Robert D. Black
Scion NeuroStim

Terese Bogucki
Decus Biomedical, LLC
Berkeley, California

Nicola Calisi
Department of Chemistry and Industrial Chemistry
University of Pisa
Pisa, Italy

Kyusun Choi
Pennsylvania State University
University Park, Pennsylvania

Ahmet F. Coskun
Electrical Engineering Department, Bioengineering Department
University of California
Los Angeles, California
and
California NanoSystems Institute
University of California
Los Angeles, California
and
Division of Chemistry and Chemical Engineering
California Institute of Technology
Pasadena, California

Daniel Filippini
Optical Devices Laboratory
IFM–Department of Physics, Chemistry and Biology
Linköping University
Linköping, Sweden

Fabio Di Francesco
Department of Chemistry and Industrial Chemistry
University of Pisa
Pisa, Italy

Flavio Griggio
Intel Corp.
Hillsboro, Oregon

Thomas N. Jackson
Pennsylvania State University
University Park, Pennsylvania

Hyunsoo Kim
Pennsylvania State University
University Park, Pennsylvania

Insoo Kim
Samsung Research America–Dallas
Richardson, Texas

Fred N. Kiwanuka
College of Computing and Information Sciences
Makerere University
Kampala, Uganda

Bernardo Melai
Department of Chemistry and Industrial Chemistry
University of Pisa
Pisa, Italy

Onur Mudanyali
Electrical Engineering Department, Bioengineering Department
University of California
Los Angeles, California
and
California NanoSystems Institute
University of California
Los Angeles, California

Ian Munabi
College of Health Sciences
Makerere University
Kampala, Uganda

Aydogan Ozcan
Electrical Engineering Department, Bioengineering Department
University of California
Los Angeles, California
and
California NanoSystems Institute
University of California
Los Angeles, California

Christian Leth Petersen
Pediatric Anesthesia Research Team
The University of British Columbia
Vancouver, Canada

Pakorn Preechaburana
Department of Physics
Faculty of Science and Technology
Thammasat University
Pathum Thani, Thailand

John A. Quinn
College of Computing and Information Sciences
Makerere University
Kampala, Uganda

Pietro Salvo
Department of Chemistry and Industrial Chemistry
University of Pisa
Pisa, Italy

Anke Suska
Optical Devices Laboratory
IFM–Department of Physics, Chemistry and Biology
Linköping University
Linköping, Sweden

Susan Trolier-McKinstry
Pennsylvania State University
University Park, Pennsylvania

Richard L. Tutwiler
Pennsylvania State University
University Park, Pennsylvania

Hongying Zhu
Electrical Engineering Department, Bioengineering Department
University of California
Los Angeles, California
and
California NanoSystems Institute
University of California
Los Angeles, California

Section 1

Sensors and Systems

1 Interfacing Diagnostics with Consumer Electronics

Pakorn Preechaburana, Anke Suska, and Daniel Filippini

CONTENTS

1.1 INTRODUCTION

The growth of ageing populations is expected to stress the demand on medical facilities in the coming decades [1]. A sensible approach to satisfy this demand is to provide essential services at hospitals while decentralizing routine diagnostics and monitoring. The challenges posed to the diagnostics platforms fitting in this scheme are numerous and diverse types of solutions are partly suitable, from point-of-care (POC) instrumentation [2,3] to simple home tests. Distinctive aspects of these solutions are the particular compromises adopted between features such as accuracy, sophistication, throughput, versatility, simplicity, mobility, and cost. Essentially, uncompromised performance at the expense of cost and mobility is typical for classical POC solutions, whereas disposable home tests for visual inspection [4] are strong in deployability and cost-effectiveness. Between these two extremes, there are emerging strategies that exploit consumer electronic devices (CEDs) as vehicles for cost-effective, sophisticated, and decentralized diagnosis.

Here we examine recent developments in these approaches and address the advantages and challenges of different implementations. CEDs such as flatbed scanners [5,6], CD/DVD drives [7–10], and computer sets with web cameras [11] have been demonstrated for chemical sensing [12] and diagnostic [13] purposes since the early 2000s. Chemical sensing solutions that operate on CEDs have the potential to reach larger populations than dedicated instruments. However, such potential has not materialized yet, and most solutions of this type operate as dedicated instruments.

One of the reasons is the need of accessory parts to interface the chemical sensing part with the CEDs. In order to provide proper analytical performance these accessory parts become specialized and constitute dedicated instrumentation themselves. Thus, although the CEDs are ubiquitous, the chemical sensing assemblies are not.

Concurrently, technological progress has sidelined some of these original CED platforms, such as the case of CD/DVD units, which are disappearing from new laptop computers, as well as separated web cameras that are now embedded in computer frames. In addition, most of the resources and implementations used for optical chemical sensing using camera/screen combinations [9–11] can be migrated to modern cellphones [14,15], which is the more appealing, truly mobile, and most pervasive CED platform. Modern cellphones, smartphones, and mobile computers (including tablets, surface PCs, and ultrabooks) also share industrial design features, such as front cameras embedded under a continuous glass sheet, which make some types of solutions compatible with all platforms. This possibility to migrate chemical sensing interfaces to different mobile platforms is also strengthened by the use of common operating systems across brands and models.

Modern advanced chemical sensing also entails sample conditioning. Micro total analysis systems (μTAS) and lab-on-a-chip (LOC) devices [16] support sample conditioning, demand small amounts of sample and reagents, and can be integrated in convenient formats for decentralized uses. LOC devices can also be disposable; however, LOC has not materialized as the most ubiquitous vehicle for distributed analysis, and one reason [17] is the lack of autonomy due to auxiliary instrumentation required for operation and readout.

Some examples of unconventional fluidics, such as 3D paper devices [18], have been shown to be suitable with simple readout; however, the migration of classic microfluidic conditioning is elusive for highly distributed scenarios. Thus, instrumentation based on CEDs concurrently offers a complementary vehicle to realize ubiquitous diagnostics using well-established classic LOC technologies.

In this chapter two distinctive approaches are addressed: CED instrumentation using permanent accessories on specific CEDs, with or without definitive modifications of the CED, and instrumentation aiming at diverse unmodified CEDs complemented by disposable devices integrating chemical sensing and readout coupling functions.

1.2 CED INSTRUMENTATION WITH ACCESSORIES

Advances in CEDs were already substantial at the beginning of the 2000s, and in particular computer peripherals were able to support chemical sensing. Starting in 2000 with the demonstration of practical colorimetric chemical sensing using flatbed scanners [6], CD and later DVD and Blu-ray drives were explored for chemical sensing uses [7,8,19]. In the case of CD/DVD drives, some demonstrations had the double role of optical readout and sample conditioning [7,20]. Also, the combination of web cameras and computer screens, used as light sources, were investigated for chemical sensing and diagnostic purposes [9–11]. The instrumentation requirements in this case are equivalent to the present capabilities of cellphones, and several of those solutions can be implemented with phones [12,13]. Examples of phenomena used in this approach include: spectral fingerprinting in transmission [9], reflection [21], and fluorescence [10,22] modes, ellipsometry [23] and surface plasmon resonance (SPR) [24], for diverse targets such as gas and odor detection [25], food analysis [10], biomarkers such as anti-neutrophil cytoplasm antibodies (ANCA) [11] and cell viability assays [9]. Measurements with flatbed scanners have been applied to gas and odor sensing [6,26], with applications demonstrated for food targets [27,28], and detection of lung cancer [29,30]. In the case of CD/DVDs used as readers, they have been demonstrated for Ca^{2+} detection [8], and diverse other targets involving biomolecular binding events [9,31], as well as detection of foodborne pathogens [32].

All these platforms have specific advantages and disadvantages, and in all cases peripherals or permanent accessory elements were used for sample conditioning and/or positioning. Flatbed scanners are capable colorimetric detectors, whereas they are difficult to exploit for other types of detection. Sample evaluation can be simple for skilled users, and elementary processing only involves image subtraction and scaling, but scanners are peripherals highly dependent on specific drivers, and periodic updates are necessary to keep up with changes in the operating systems. Development of customized chemical sensing applications, for general users, thus becomes hampered by the diversity of brands and models that should be supported. Therefore, although chemical sensing with scanners is based on CED platforms, they are normally operated as dedicated instruments. Finally, the bulky scanner format restricts mobile uses.

Figure 1.1a shows the scanner evaluation of a colorimetric sensing array with 11 functional materials, which selectively change color upon exposure to different analytes, thus creating response patterns that identify chemical species. The same principle was used with a 36 elements array for the detection of volatiles in exhaled air, linked to the identification of lung cancer [29].

CD/DVD drives constitute compact interferometers operating with laser light, in a configuration designed to resolve nanometric features. Several optical phenomena are in principle measurable with this platform [8]; however, it has mostly been exploited for reflectance and absorbance [7–9,30,31]. The CD/DVD drives also offer the possibility to implement sample conditioning by controlling the centrifugal forces on fluids within fluidics integrated CDs [7,33]. The major drawback of this platform, for temporary use as a chemical sensing reader, is the difficulty to control the CD readout only by software. CD/DVD drives write/read information in coded locations not easily accessible at high-level programing, and the actual solutions are dedicated instruments with the required hardware interfacing [34]. Furthermore, although they contain a laser light source, or more than one in DVD/Blu-ray devices [34], the choice of absorption transduced chemical responses is restricted to the few available spectral windows.

Figure 1.1b shows a DVD readout system applied to the detection of Ca^{+2} ions in solution. A chemically sensitive functional material was applied as multiple tracks on the DVD surface. The tracks were exposed to increasing concentrations of Ca^{+2}, and the sensing material optically responded with increasing absorbance within the laser spectral window. Software and hardware interfacing enables the readout of such responses and dedicated post-processing complements an analytical resolution compatible with quantitative analyses.

Alternatively to this type of hardware implementation, there are also examples aiming at only software readout, where the reading error statistic of chemically functionalized CDs is monitored as an indicator of CD status before and after exposure to analytes [35]. This error rate is accessible by software. Flatbed scanners and CD/DVD units are not standalone CEDs but computer peripherals, and in both cases require associated computers to operate.

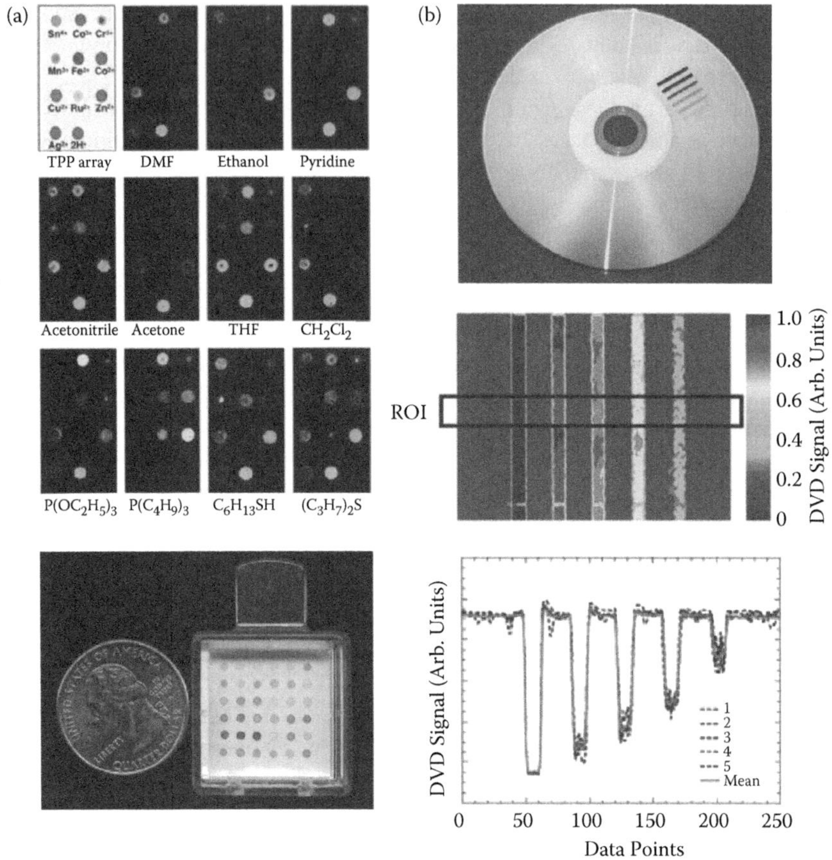

FIGURE 1.1 (a) Color response patterns of a metalloporphyrin sensor array. The images were subtracted (absolute value) from the initial array image using Adobe Photoshop®. (Reprinted from N. Rakow, K. Suslick, A colorimetric sensor array for odour visualization, *Nature* 406, 2000, 710–713. With permission from Macmillan.) Colorimetric sensor array used for lung cancer detection, consisting of 36 chemically sensitive dots on a disposable sensor. (Reprinted from P. Mazzone et al. Lung cancer diagnosis by the analysis of exhaled breath with a colorimetric sensor array. *Thorax* 62, 2007, 565–568. With permission from BMJ.) (b) Implementation of lab-on-DVD for quantitative analysis. Photograph of a conventional DVD with a reference gray scale pattern quantification of the sensor response. False-color image of the scanned gray scale pattern with a region of interest (ROI) employed for further signal enhancement. The mean from the ROI intensities is used for quantification. (Reprinted from R. Potyrailo et al. Analog signal acquisition from computer optical disk drives for quantitative chemical sensing, *Anal. Chem.* 78, 2006, 5893–5899. With permission from American Chemical Society.) *(continued)*

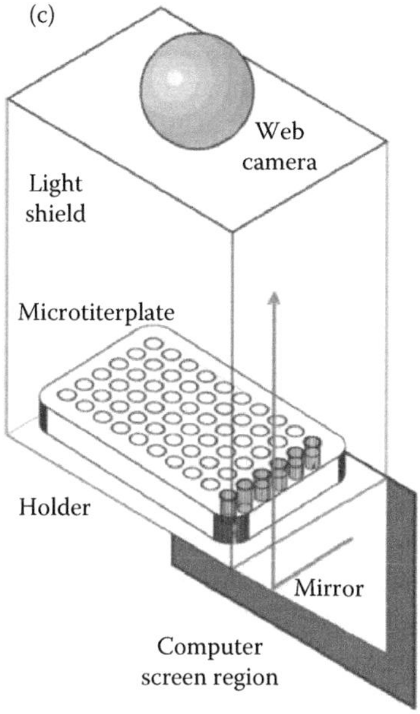

FIGURE 1.1 (CONTINUED) (c) Diagram of the experimental setup used in ELISA plate detection of ANCA. A region of a computer screen provided a color sequence that illuminated a microtiter plate from below, with the help of a mirror. The microtiter plate was placed in a removable holder that also provided a light shield from ambient light and supported the web camera. A video stream of the assay was captured and processed for quantification. (Reprinted from D. Filippini, K. Tejle, I. Lundström, ELISA test for anti-neutrophil cytoplasm antibodies detection evaluated by a computer screen photo-assisted technique, *Biosensors and Bioelectronics* 21, 2005, 266–272. With permission from Elsevier.)

In the case of systems that use computer screens as light sources and web cameras as detectors, the peripherals are nowadays highly integrated in single units, such as in phones, laptops, and tablets. One key advantage of this CED assembly is the versatility of the screens used as light sources. Numerous types of image formats are universally supported and controlling screen color, intensity, patterns, and pattern location in 2D coordinates is easily implemented on any of these devices by just displaying designed images, without the need to develop specific drivers or advanced programming.

After display control, image acquisition is the simplest action to command, and the combination with the light source embedded in a same device makes the concept attractive for compact instrumentation. Limitations of this approach are related to the light source intensity and readout image quality, especially with early types of detectors.

Similarly to the other types of CED instrumentation, permanent accessory parts were used to align and hold chemically sensitive interfaces in place, between the light source and the imager [11–13]. Figure 1.1c shows the schematics of a sample holder used for a 96-well microplates readout using a computer screen as light source. This arrangement was used for diverse sensing targets, and in this particular reference corresponds to an ELISA assay for anti-neutrophil cytoplasmatic antibodies (ANCA), a biomarker used for the diagnostics of bowel inflammatory disease [13].

Permanent accessory parts, as those considered in previous examples, enable efficient control of the measuring conditions and accelerate the development of concrete solutions; however, they restrict the ubiquity of the CEDs. A major attraction of instrumentation on CEDs is the large availability of these devices, whereas systems that require specialized accessories are only as ubiquitous as the accessory and essentially as rare as any computer interfaced instrument.

Cell phones are today the natural choice of CED measuring platform due to their ubiquity, sophistication, and processing power, which surpasses, in some cases the capabilities of computers in early demonstrations of CED instrumentation [11].

Chemical sensing using cellphones has been demonstrated with the phones embedded as a permanent part of the instrumentation, and used for communication and processing purposes. An example of this is the monitoring of urban pollution in gas phase [36]. The concept uses mobile internet devices and cellphones to capture, process, and disseminate sensor data, in scenarios where sensor infrastructure is not available and geographic mapping of pollution is required. Devices such as those in Figure 1.2a were conceived for air quality sensing on street sweepers and support collection of CO, NO_x, O_3, temperature, and humidity data.

Other examples involve electronic interfacing to dedicated chemical sensing arrays operating with a specific cellphone model [37]. In this case the cellphone can be disconnected from the chemical sensing accessory and still be utilized for its regular purpose (Figure 1.2b).

In the past few years, optical instrumentation, such as a microscope, has been associated to cellphones, where the phone provided a camera and the possibility of remote assessment and diagnostic by an expert [38]. Platforms like these are capable of identifying malaria and sickle cell anemia in bright field (Figure 1.2c), and *Mycobacterium tuberculosis* in infected sputum samples in fluorescence mode. As expected, fluorescence imaging requires intense illumination and the microscope to incorporate its own light source.

Simpler configurations using fixed spherical lenses and micro-positioning for the specimen have also been demonstrated with cellphone cameras, and at 1.5 μm resolution this is shown to be compatible with cell analysis for diagnostics [39]. Figure 1.2d shows the cross-section of a stained stem structure imaged in bright field with a regular microscope and using the phone. The ultimate resolution can be achieved by combining multiple focal images from a micro-positioned sample. Although these solutions are specific to the phones used, no permanent modifications are introduced in the CED and upon disassembly from the instrument the phone camera is still usable.

Holographic lensfree microscopy has also recently been demonstrated on cellphones [40–43] (Figure 1.2e). In this case the phone lens must be removed, making the instrumentation permanent. Several diagnostic targets have been demonstrated with these platforms, including density of white blood cells, red blood cells, hemoglobin [41], and allergens [44].

Cardiac markers such as NT-proBNP are routinely used to monitor patients with heart failure [45,46]. Established commercial tests exist, which are based on lateral flow devices and immune-detection, and provide quantitative contrast responses that can be read by dedicated instruments. This type of readout using cellphones has also

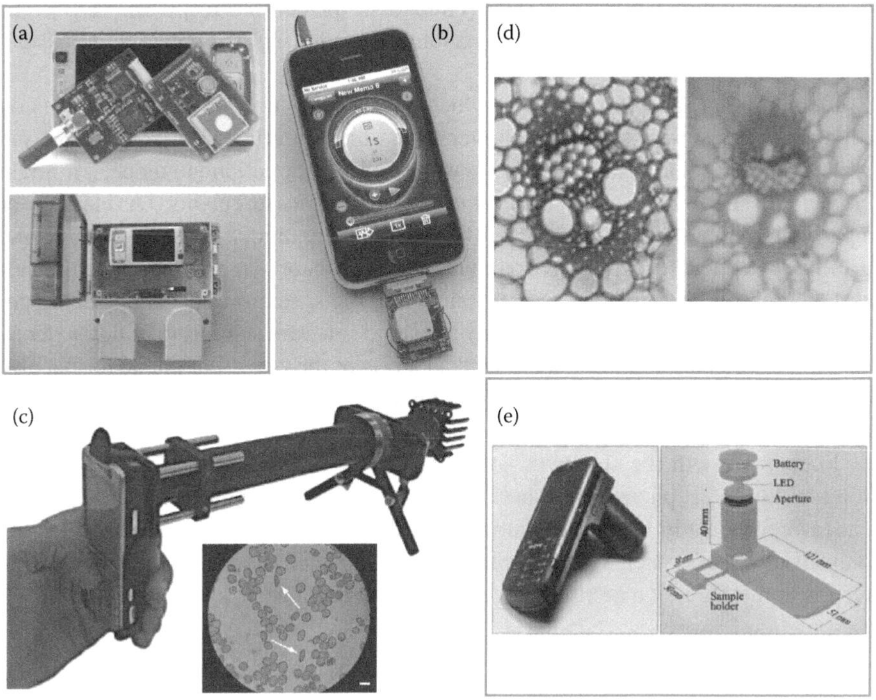

FIGURE 1.2 (a) Phone enabled carbon monoxide (CO), nitrogen oxide (NOx), and ozone (O_3) gas sensors as well as temperature, relative humidity, and motion (3D accelerometer) sensors. Location data is provided via GPS on the integrated mobile phone. (Reprinted from P.M. Aoki et al. Common Sense: Mobile Environmental Sensing Platforms to Support Community Action and Citizen Science. *Adjunct Proceedings Ubicomp* 2008, Sep. 2008, 59–60, under the open access license by the School of Computer Science at Research Showcase. With permission.) (b) Multiple-channel silicon-based sensing chip, which consists of 64 nanosensors. The chemical sensing prototype is plugged into an iPhone 30-pin dock connector. (Reprinted from J. Li, Cell Phone Chemical Sensor, 2009, NASA Ames Research Center. With permission.) (c) Mobile phone microscopy, and sample image. This prototype, with filters and LED illumination is capable of fluorescence imaging. Mobile phone microscopy images of diseased blood smear with sickle-cell anemia. (Reprinted from D. Breslauer et al. Mobile phone based clinical microscopy for global health applications, *PLoS ONE* 4, 2009, e6320, under the Creative Commons Attribution License. With permission.) (d) Cell phone microscope with 1mm diameter ball lens in front of the cellphone camera system. Commercial microscope image of stained plant stems (left) compared with the cellphone result (right). (Reprinted from Z. Smith et al. Cell-phone-based platform for biomedical device development and education applications, *PLoS ONE* 6, 2011, e17150, under the Creative Commons Attribution License. With permission.) (e) Lensfree cellphone microscope. The additional gadget installed on the cellphone integrates a light emitting diode and an aperture. The samples are loaded from the side through a mechanical sample holder. (Reprinted from D. Tseng et al. Lensfree microscopy on a cellphone, *Lab Chip* 10, 2010, 1787–1792. With permission from The Royal Society of Chemistry.)

been demonstrated. In this case phone screens are used as controlled light sources to compose high dynamic range (HDR) images of the contrast response [14,47]. The HDR technique doubles the analytical resolution, and brings the phone camera capabilities within the diagnostics range.

It could be argued that solutions which do not introduce permanent changes on cellphones are more attractive; however, given the fast renewal of cellphones, and that temporary solutions are bound anyway to particular cellphone models, it might not be an issue to dedicate a replaced cellphone for measurements. Developing for a particular phone model implies, on the other hand, a unique accessory design and a fully controlled software environment. The continuous upgrading of cellphones and the consolidation of two main phone operating systems, and vibrant developer communities, introduces the possibility to extend software support to multiple phone generations. In addition, the generalized adoption of the candy bar phone format also contributes to some level of standardization and consequently accessories would fit to more than one phone model.

In contrast with the strategies surveyed in this section, the design of a generic solution fitting all phone types and models is a more demanding and less explored endeavor, especially when the solution should not imply permanent accessories but only disposable elements deployable at the same scale as the phones. Emerging results in this direction are the subject of the next section.

1.3 CED INSTRUMENTATION WITHOUT PERMANENT ACCESSORIES

Popular disposable devices for diagnostics, such as pregnancy test strips [48] are commonly simple enough to be evaluated by visual inspection. This type of implementation can be extended to semi quantitative categories in urine tests [49] and for the detection of many chemical substances [50]. Quantitative detection normally requires complementary readers, which are specific for each test and brand [49].

Depending on the application and user needs, dedicated readers can be acceptable, such as in the case of routine glucose monitoring [51] required by diabetic patients, whereas in other situations the reader is an obstacle. Furthermore, some readers are not conceived to be deployable, for example, in quantitative disposable tests, such as those used for cardiac markers (NT-proBNP, Troponin T, Myoglobin, D-Dimer) [52], or multiparameter urine test strips [53], which utilize dedicated point-of-care readers at medical care centers.

Modern LOC based solutions for diagnostics [3,54–57] are normally implemented as POC instruments, and are conceived to operate in specialized environments. Bringing the sophistication of LOC solutions outside the medical environment is challenging and stresses the demands on readers' availability and cost. Alternatives to classic LOC, such as paper fluidics (Figure 1.3a), have been proposed and demonstrated for colorimetric detection evaluated with phone cameras [18,58]. An important aspect demonstrated in this work is also the embedded calibrations designed in the fluidics, which is crucial for detections where the illumination cannot be controlled, and a fresh reference acquired with each evaluation makes the technique more robust.

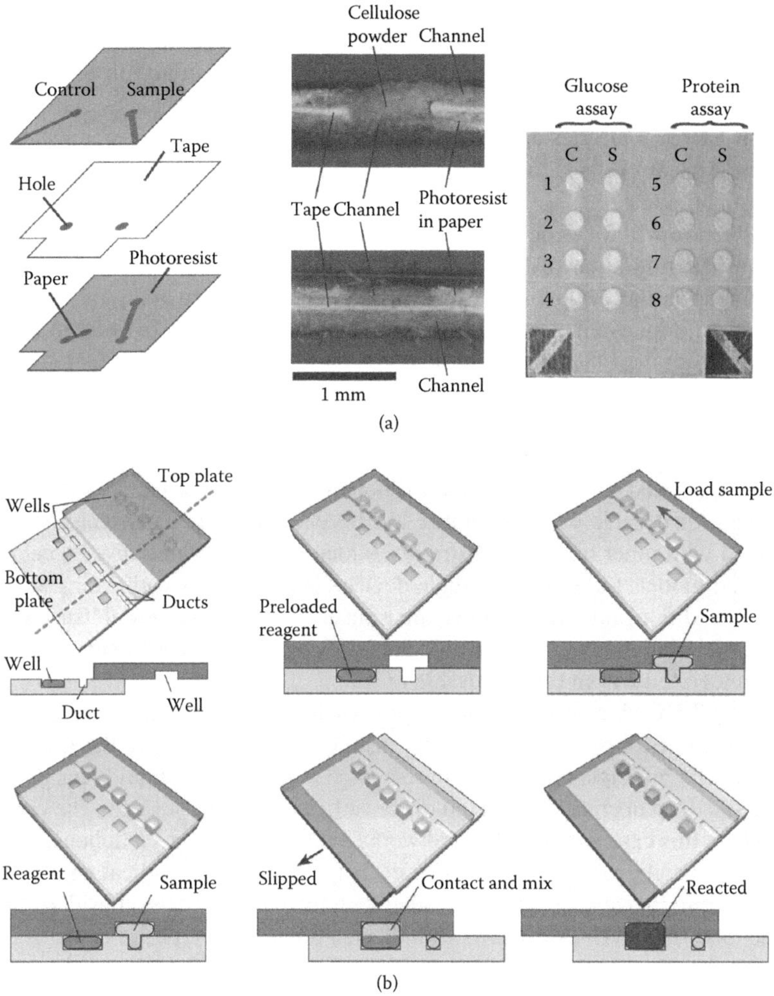

FIGURE 1.3 (a) 3D paper fluidics showing a module consisting of paper channels confined with photoresist (light gray) and separated between multiple levels through holes punched on double-sided adhesive tape (white layer). The cross section shows the connection and the insulation between different levels. Example of parallel assays with integrated controls. (Reprinted from A. Martinez, S. Phillips, G. Whitesides, Three-dimensional microfluidic devices fabricated in layered paper and tape, *PNAS* 105, 2008, 19606–19611. With permission from National Academy of Sciences, United States.) (b) Step-by-step 3D schematic drawings with cross-section views describing the operation of the SlipChip concept. Preloaded wells of the bottom plate, and the channels of the bottom plate, are connected in sequence to the upper plate when they slip on. View of the device with top and bottom plates aligned. Loading of a single sample by overlapping channels of the bottom plate and wells of the top plate. Slipping of the top plate relative to the bottom plate disconnects the sample wells of the top plate from the channels of the bottom plate (lower row), thus exposing the sample wells to the reagents. The dark gray well indicates a reaction taking place after mixing and incubation. (Reprinted from W. Du et al. SlipChip, *Lab Chip* 9, 2009, 2286–2292. With permission from The Royal Society of Chemistry.)

Further progress on the fluidics, aiming at more sophisticated detection schemes and sequential sample conditioning, has also been shown through the introduction of slip chip approaches [59], which have also been demonstrated in paper fluidics [60] (Figure 1.3b). These technologies entail different performances and versatilities from LOC on plastics and glass, which constitute a vast legacy of established solutions. A clear obstacle to exploit the classic LOCs is the lack of ubiquitous light sources and readout.

This section will focus on recent demonstrations addressing these challenges and aiming at the migration of classical LOC technologies to CEDs' evaluation. The first example is the evaluation of disposable LOC microstructures on cellphones. The problem implies imaging the detection region of the LOC. In order to keep the device compact the LOC device must be at a close distance to the camera, but cellphone cameras are not designed to focus at few millimeters from the camera surface, and thus a refocusing element becomes necessary.

Recent solutions using permanent elements and specimen micro-positioning have been demonstrated for microscopy on iPhone devices [39], whereas solutions just involving a disposable element require a different approach. This scenario can be completed with other relevant constraints, which include serving diverse cellphone brands and models rather than a single device, and making it with a single generic design. In addition, although adaptive focusing elements are well-established devices [61–63], the solution in this case should not imply a permanent accessory, but a component integrated within the disposable LOC.

Imaging LOC elements at about 50-μm resolution implies moderate magnification and the optical performance should just be enough to observe the LOC detection area. The principle considered in reference [64] utilizes a liquid lens produced by a sessile drop operating at a fixed distance from the LOC surface. The complete assembly in this case is disposable and works in principle on any cellphone, not even requiring specialized acquisition software but the standard applications for video and time-lapse image acquisition provided with the phones. In the considered example, the focusing device was tested with diverse brands and types of cameras across different generations and operating systems, which include Symbian, iOS, and Mac OS X controlled devices.

Central to this solution is the generic design of the device; the same fixed configuration fits all CED platforms. The operating principle consists of a liquid drop on a Polydimethylsiloxane (PDMS) membrane sitting on the camera surface. This disposable membrane provides sufficient adhesion to the camera surface, and can be gently removed after use. In addition, it provides optical matching between the back of the drop and the camera, and finally it incorporates a circular depression to confine the drop to the center of the viewing field (Figure 1.4a). The PDMS contributes the necessary surface energy to condition the sessile drop contact angle, which defines the curvature and thus the lens's back focal length. The rest of the structure is a 2 mm PDMS separator holding the glass substrate with the LOC fluidics. During operation the lens evaporates changing the back focal length in a broad range that can cover most focal variations existing across camera brands and models (Figure 1.4b). Time-lapse acquisition with the cellphone enables focus identification and evaluation of experiments run within the LOC fluidics (Figure 1.4c). The considered 400-μm

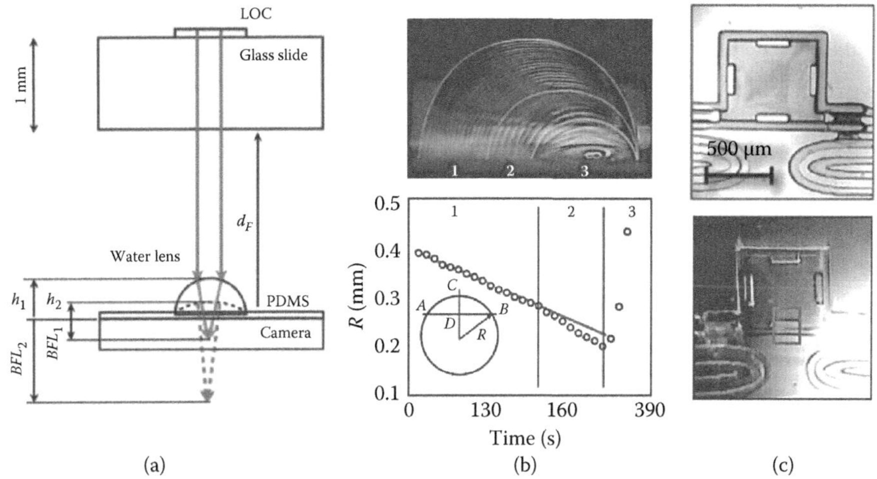

FIGURE 1.4 (a) Cross section of the measuring device. The liquid lens is represented at two different volumes with the associated back focal lengths (*BFL*). The forward distance (d_F) is 1 and 2 mm in the experiments and it is defined by PDMS structural elements. (b) Collection of sessile drop images captured with a stereomicroscope at a 15s interval. The evaporation regimes (indicated as 1, 2, and 3) are highlighted; characterization of the drop evaporation by the drop radius of curvature, calculated from measured chord and height distances at 15s intervals. (c) 100X magnifications of the LOC chamber imaged with an Axiovert 40 inverted microscope and with an iSight camera with the disposable adaptive lens. (Reprinted from P. Preechaburana, A. Suska, D. Filippini, Embedded adaptive optics for ubiquitous lab-on-a-chip readout on intact cell phones, *Sensors* 12, 2012, 8586–8600, under the Creative Commons Attribution License. With permission.)

radius lens enables a back focal length scanning between 500 μm and 4 mm and different magnifications can be achieved depending on the set front distance.

Evaporating conditions, PDMS preparation, and surface conditioning determine the regime through which the sessile drop evaporates. Sessile drop evaporation is a complex non-stationary phenomenon inducing well-defined geometric transitions during the evaporation. Three different regimes can be observed for the present configuration. In the first regime (1 in Figure 1.4b), occurring for about half of the recorded time, the contact angle remains practically constant and the evaporation changes the drop curvature by reducing the chord and height. In the second regime (2 in Figure 1.4b) the process accelerates, which can be noticed by the larger spacing between captures, and a noticeable change in contact angle, while the drop chord and height keep changing. In the third and last regime (3 in Figure 1.4b), the changes accelerate, but the drop is pinned at a constant chord and only the contact angle and drop height changes. The considered lens is used in the third regime, although the other modes are possible, exploiting the slower focal changes compatible with assays that demand longer response times.

The migration of advanced detection methods to disposable devices, which operate on CED platforms, is central to consolidate this strategy. Concurrently, the use of generic detection methods that can be sensitized to diverse targets contributes to standardize and simplify usage.

Surface plasmon resonance (SPR) [65] is a benchmark for biosensing and affinity analysis. SPR is also a generic method, which can be tailored for diverse target analytes through surface functionalization. In addition, the technique is compatible with label-free analysis, which contributes to its specificity and to simpler sample conditioning schemes. In SPR visible photons are conditioned to excite a plasmon that propagates at a metal insulator interface. The result of this resonant energy transfer is a characteristic dip in the reflected intensity versus photon momentum and energy. The coordinates of this dip are highly sensitive to surface conditions and can be used to transduce biorecognition events, such as ligand interaction between an antigen and a surface functionalized with a complementary antibody.

SPR systems are normally configured as laboratory equipment [64,66–69], although compact instruments [70,71] and SPR modules [72] have also been demonstrated. Designing SPR as a disposable element that transforms any unmodified cellphone into an SPR reader implies a number of challenges. In the first place, an optical coupler for total internal reflection is required in SPR measurements, and it has to be fabricated in disposable materials such as PDMS. This optical coupler captures light from the phone screen and conditions the illumination on a thin Au film, which is the vehicle of the SPR phenomenon. For detection in aqueous solutions, the PDMS optics conditions the illumination between 67° and 77°, which is suitable to capture the SPR dip in Au for red and green light, both simply provided by setting the phone screen color (Figure 1.5a and b). Reflected light is then guided to produce an image on the cellphone camera, and software in the phone commands a time-lapse acquisition to capture standard SPR sensorgrams. The concept is compatible with regular LOC technology and PDMS fluidics, which sit atop of the Au surface (Figure 1.5c).

SPR features a number of convenient aspects for implementation on CEDs. A first favorable aspect is that light source intensity is not determinant in the sensitivity, such as in the case of fluorescence measurements, which normally require an accessory light source [41]. Accordingly, the 300 to 500 cd/m^2 available from any phone screen suffices to perform SPR detection, contributing to the SPR implementation based solely on a disposable element.

A second remarkable characteristic of angle-resolved SPR detection is that the limited camera dynamic range does not restrict the technique resolution, and any phone camera can capture the contrast levels generated in the SPR measurement. Upon processing, quantification is related to the spatial resolution and localization of the SPR dip. Regular front cameras have 640 × 480 pixel resolution at least, which surpasses the 8 bit/channel (256 levels) bound to intensity detection. Typical characterization with known refractive index solutions shows a resolution of 2.14×10^{-6} RIU, which compares well with commercial SPR modules (1×10^{-6} RIU) [71].

The platform was tested for the detection of β_2 microglobulin (Figure 1.6), a well-established biomarker for cancer, inflammatory disorders, and kidney disease [73–75]. Sensorgrams using a commercial Biacore CM5 dextran surface chip functionalized for β_2 microglobulin, are shown in Figure 1.6. The limit of detection (LOD) for label-free conditioning is 0.1 μg/mL. Considering normal values in

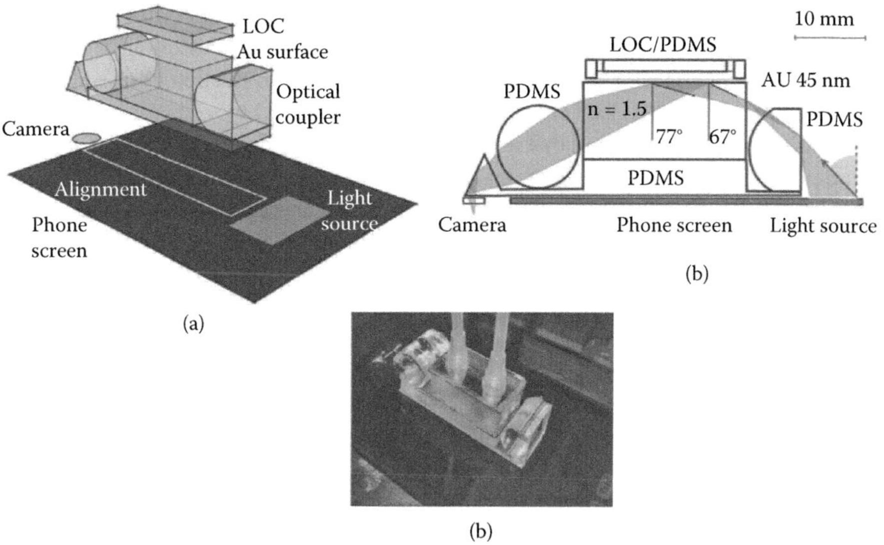

FIGURE 1.5 (a) 3D scheme of a representative setup for angle-resolved SPR using screen illumination and front camera detection optically coupled by a disposable device. (b) 2D raytrace of the experimental arrangement showing the light path from screen to camera. (c) Picture of the actual experimental arrangement. (Reprinted from P. Preechaburana et al. Surface plasmon resonance chemical sensing on cell phones, *Angew. Chem. Int. Ed.* 51, 2012, 11585–11588. With permission from Wiley-VCH Verlag GmbH.)

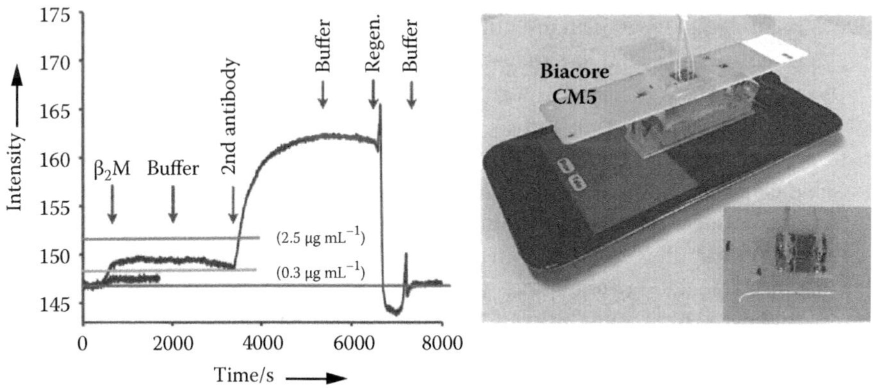

FIGURE 1.6 Interaction analysis of a commercial Biacore CM5 test chip functionalized for β_2 microglobulin detection and tested at 1.32 μg mL^{-1} and 0.132 μg mL^{-1} concentrations. The baseline of the measurement is indicated with lines corresponding to normal serum (< 2.5 μg mL^{-1}) and urine (< 0.3 μg mL^{-1}) levels, respectively. (Reprinted from P. Preechaburana et al. Surface plasmon resonance chemical sensing on cell phones, *Angew. Chem. Int. Ed.* 51, 2012, 11585–11588. With permission from Wiley-VCH Verlag GmbH.)

plasma of 2.5 μg/mL [73] the concept is suitable with β_2 microglobulin monitoring. For this LOD the concept is also compatible with label-free detection in urine, in which the normal level is 0.3 μg/mL. In both cases the introduction of an amplification antibody brings the LOD to the ng/mL range (Figure 1.6).

This demonstration shows that a purely disposable solution, with a single configuration can operate with sufficient analytical performance on unmodified cellphones (iOS, Android, and Symbian platforms of diverse generations were tested in this work) [15]. Furthermore, the concept is compatible with classical LOC fluidics and sample conditioning, which represents a vast legacy of well-crafted solutions that can be thus migrated to cellphones.

The ultimate implementation does certainly require an entirely autonomous LOC (ALOC) [76] sample conditioning. Emerging examples of ALOC are promising [77,78], and further progress on this aspect will be required to materialize ALOC on a phone. Recent progress on controlled priming [79], passive fluidics [80–82], and slip chip [58] technologies, add to the toolbox of suitable alternatives that can complete all the necessary requirements to materialize autonomous disposable LOC readable on CEDs, in the near future.

1.4 CONCLUSIONS

Interfacing diagnostics with CEDs is a sensible strategy to exploit the residual capacity of available, sophisticated, and continuously evolving infrastructure. Aside from physical parameters, medical diagnostics entangles quantitative chemical sensing and thus it constitutes an elusive target for decentralization. Chemical sensing implies multivocal stimuli able to produce a response, and at the same time detection involves some degree of reaction and deterioration of the functional materials. In comparison with specific physical sensors univocally responding, for instance, to acceleration or magnetic field direction, reusable chemical sensing is more demanding, less autonomous, and less robust.

A common strategy, clearly reflected in CEDs interfacing, is the adoption of single-use sensing elements instead of reusable devices. Most examples in this work illustrate this option. Single-use sensors, which are consequently conceived as disposable elements, allow for more specific chemical recognition of target analytes. At the same time disposability eliminates maintenance and periodic calibration, and ultimately it simplifies usage, a key aspect considering the decentralization promised by this instrumentation paradigm.

Nevertheless, the disposability of sensing elements does not grant direct exploitation of CEDs for robust readout. As shown in this review, diverse adaptors and sample holders providing different alternatives to couple sensing elements to the CEDs have been explored. While considering the ubiquity of CEDs, and specially cellphones, as a central motivation for this technology, it seems evident that the CED/adaptor set is only as ubiquitous as the adaptor, and typically rare compared with the CEDs.

Specific sample coupler designs, fitting to a particular phone model, or implying permanent modification on the phones, have been shown as well-performing dedicated instruments, but at the expense of a significantly restricted ubiquity.

Innovative solutions exploiting the autonomy of disposable paper fluidics and integrating embedded calibration for quantitative readout, demonstrates a concept with the potential to match the ubiquity of cellphones. On the other hand, unconventional LOC technology cannot fully migrate the strong legacy of sophisticated and diverse solutions existing for glass and plastic LOC.

A final concept aiming at conventional LOC technology integrated in disposable couplers, and able to deliver LOC analytical performance has been considered. This approach aims at marrying conventional LOC analytical prowess with CED's instrumentation ubiquity, while incorporating design features to support evaluation across phone or mobile computing models and brands, indistinctly, with a single sensor design.

Some promising examples of this approach have been illustrated in this work. Further progress in this direction will require the complete integration of sample conditioning in an autonomous disposable LOC. Emerging examples of semi-autonomous and sequential sample conditioning suggest that the ultimate materialization of ubiquitous LOC diagnostics on CEDs is not only promising but also feasible.

REFERENCES

1. R. Gossink and J. Souquet, Advances and Trends in Health Care Technology, Chapter 1, in *Advances in Healthcare Technology, Shaping the Future of Medical Care*, Philips Research Book Series, Vol. 6, G. Spekowius and T. Wendler (Eds.), Springer, Dordrecht, The Netherlands, 2006.
2. N. Pant Pai, C. Vadnais, C. Denkinger, N. Engel, M. Pai, Point-of-care testing for infectious diseases: Diversity, complexity, and barriers in low- and middle-income countries, *PLOS Medicine* 09, 2012, e1001306.
3. V. Gubala, L.F. Harris, A.J. Ricco, M.X. Tan, D.E. Williams, Point of care diagnostics: Status and future, *Anal. Chem.* 84, 2012, 487–515.
4. J. Ehrenkranz, Home and point-of-care pregnancy tests: A review of the technology, *Epidemiology* 13, 2002, 3S.
5. W. Hruschka, D. Massie, J. Anderson, Computerized analysis of two-dimensional electrophoretograms, *Anal. Chem.* 55, 1983, 2345–2348.
6. N. Rakow, K. Suslick, A colorimetric sensor array for odour visualization, *Nature* 406, 2000, 710–713.
7. D. Duffy, H. Gillis, J. Lin, N. Sheppard, G. Kellogg, Microfabricated centrifugal microfluidic systems: Characterization and multiple enzymatic assays, *Anal. Chem.* 71, 1999, 4669–4678.
8. S. Lai, S. Wang, J. Luo, L. Lee, S. Yang, M. Madou, Design of a compact disk-like microfluidic platform for enzyme-linked immunosorbent assay, *Anal. Chem.* 76, 2004, 1832–1837.
9. R. Potyrailo, W. Morris, A. Leach, T. Sivavec, M. Wisnudel, S. Boyette, Analog signal acquisition from computer optical disk drives for quantitative chemical sensing, *Anal. Chem.* 78, 2006, 5893–5899.
10. S. Lange, G. Roth, S. Wittemann, T. Lacoste, A. Vetter, J. Grässle, S. Kopta, M. Kolleck, B. Breitinger, M. Wick, J. Hörber, S. Dübel, A. Bernard, Measuring biomolecular binding events with a compact disc player device, *Angew. Chem. Int. Ed.* 45, 2006, 270–273.
11. D. Filippini, S. Svensson, L. Lundström, Computer screen as a programmable light source for visible absorption characterization of (bio)chemical assays, *Chem. Comm.* 2, 2003, 240–241.

12. D. Filippini, A. Alimelli, C. Di Natale, R. Paolesse, A. D'Amico, I. Lundström, Chemical sensing with familiar devices, *Angew. Chem. Int. Ed.* 45, 2006, 3800–3803.
13. D. Filippini, K. Tejle, I. Lundström, ELISA test for anti-neutrophil cytoplasm antibodies detection evaluated by a computer screen photo-assisted technique, *Biosens. Bioelectro.* 21, 2005, 266–272.
14. P. Preechaburanaa, S. Macken, A. Suska, D. Filippini, HDR imaging evaluation of a NT-proBNP test with a mobile phone, *Biosens. Bioelectro.* 26, 2011, 2107–2113.
15. P. Preechaburana, M. Collado Gonzalez, A. Suska, D. Filippini, Surface plasmon resonance chemical sensing on cell phones, *Angew. Chem. Int. Ed.* 51, 2012, 11585–11588.
16. V.F. Cardoso, G. Minas, Micro Total Analysis Systems, Chapter 11, in *Microfluidics and Nanofluidics Handbook; Fabrication, Implementation, and Applications*, S. Mitra, S. Chakraborty (Eds.), Boca Raton: CRC Press, 2012.
17. G. Whitesides, The origins and the future of microfluidics, *Nature* 442, 2006, 368–373.
18. A. Martinez, S. Phillips, G. Whitesides, Three-dimensional microfluidic devices fabricated in layered paper and tape, *PNAS* 105, 2008, 19606–19611.
19. R. Potyrailo, Ubiquitous Devices for Chemical Sensing, in *Autonomous Sensor Networks: Collective Sensing Strategies for Analytical Purposes*, D. Filippini (Ed.), Springer Series on Chemical Sensors and Biosensors (Series Ed. G. Urban), Volume 13, 2013, pp. 237–264.
20. M. Amasia, M. Cozzens, M. Madou, Centrifugal microfluidic platform for rapid PCR amplification using integrated thermoelectric heating and ice-valving, *Sensors and Actuators* B 161, 2012, 1191–1197.
21. D. Filippini, G. Comina, I. Lundström, Computer screen photo-assisted reflectance fingerprinting, *Sensors and Actuators* B 107, 2005, 580–586.
22. E. Gatto, M. Malik, C. Di Natale, R. Paolesse, A. D'Amico, I. Lundström, D. Filippini, Polychromatic fingerprinting of excitation emission matrices, *Chem. Eur. J.* 14, 2008, 6057–6060.
23. J. Bakker, H. Arwin, I. Lundström, D. Filippini, Computer screen photoassisted off-null ellipsometry, *Applied Optics* 45, 2006, 7795–7799.
24. D. Filippini, F. Winquist, I. Lundström, Computer screen photo-excited surface plasmon resonance imaging, *Analytica Chimica Acta* 625, 2008, 207–214.
25. A. Alimelli, G. Pennazza, M. Santonico, R. Paolesse, D. Filippini, A. D'Amico, I. Lundström, C. Di Natale, Fish freshness detection by a computer screen photoassisted based gas sensor array, *Analytica Chimica Acta* 582, 2007, 320–328.
26. S. Lim, L. Feng, J. Kemling, C. Musto, K. Suslick, An optoelectronic nose for the detection of toxic gases, *Nature Chemistry* 1, 2009, 562–567.
27. B. Suslick, L. Feng, K. Suslick, Discrimination of complex mixtures by a colorimetric sensor array: Coffee aromas, *Anal. Chem.* 82, 2010, 2067–2073.
28. C. Musto, S. Lim, K. Suslick, Colorimetric detection and identification of natural and artificial sweeteners, *Anal. Chem.* 81, 2009, 6526–6533.
29. P. Mazzone, J. Hammel, R. Dweik, J. Na, C. Czich, D. Laskowski, T. Mekhail, Lung cancer diagnosis by the analysis of exhaled breath with a colorimetric sensor array. *Thorax.* 62, 2007, 565–568.
30. P. Mazzone, X. Wang, Y. Xu, T. Mekhail, M. Beukemann, J. Na, J. Kemling, K. Suslick, M. Sasidhar, Exhaled breath analysis with a colorimetric sensor array for the identification and characterization of lung cancer. *Journal of Thoracic Oncology* 7, 2012, 137–142.
31. S. Morais, J. Carrascosa, D. Mira, R. Puchades, Á. Maquieira, Microimmunoanalysis on standard compact discs to determine low abundant compounds, *Anal. Chem.* 79, 2007, 7628–7635.

32. T. Arnandis-Chover, S. Morais, L. Tortajada-Genaro, R. Puchades, A. Maquieira, J. Berganza, G. Olabarria, Detection of food-borne pathogens with DNA arrays on disk, *Talanta* 101, 2012, 405–412.
33. J. Steigert, M. Grumann, T. Brenner, L. Riegger, J. Harter, R. Zengerleab, J. Ducre, Fully integrated whole blood testing by real-time absorption measurement on a centrifugal platform, *Lab Chip* 6, 2006, 1040–1044.
34. R. Potyrailo, W. Morris, R. Wroczynski, L. Hassib, P. Miller, B. Dworken, A. Leach, S. Boyette, C. Xiao, Multi-wavelength operation of optical disk drives for chemical and biological analysis, *Sensors and Actuators* B 136, 2009, 203–208.
35. Y. Li, L. Ou, H. Yu, Digitized molecular diagnostics: Reading disk-based bioassays with standard computer drives, *Anal. Chem.* 80, 2008, 8216–8223.
36. P.M. Aoki, R.J. Honicky, A. Mainwaring, C. Myers, E. Paulos, S. Subramanian, and A. Woodruff, Common Sense: Mobile Environmental Sensing Platforms to Support Community Action and Citizen Science. *Adjunct Proceedings Ubicomp* 2008, Sep. 2008, 59–60.
37. J. Li, Cell Phone Chemical Sensor, 2009, NASA Ames Research Center, http://www.nasa.gov/centers/ames/news/features/2009/cell_phone_sensors.html.
38. D. Breslauer, R. Maamari, N. Switz, W. Lam, D. Fletcher, Mobile phone based clinical microscopy for global health applications, *PLoS ONE* 4, 2009, e6320.
39. Z. Smith, K. Chu, A. Espenson, M. Rahimzadeh, A. Gryshuk, M. Molinaro, D. Dwyre, S. Lane, D. Matthews, S. Wachsmann-Hogiu, Cell-phone-based platform for biomedical device development and education applications, *PLoS ONE* 6, 2011, e17150.
40. D. Tseng, O. Mudanyali, C. Oztoprak, S. Isikman, I. Sencan, O. Yaglidere, A. Ozcan, Lensfree microscopy on a cellphone, *Lab Chip* 10, 2010, 1787–1792.
41. S. Isikman, W. Bishara, O. Mudanyali, I. Sencan, T. Su, D. Tseng, O. Yaglidere, U. Sikora, A. Ozcan, Lensfree on-chip microscopy and tomography for biomedical applications, *IEEE J. of Selected Topics in Quantum Electronics* 18, 2012, 1059–1072.
42. H. Zhu, S. Isikman, O. Mudanyali, A. Greenbaum, A. Ozcan, Optical imaging techniques for point-of-care diagnostics, *Lab Chip* 13, 2013, 51–67.
43. H. Zhu, I. Sencan, J. Wong, S. Dimitrov, D. Tseng, K. Nagashimaa, A. Ozcan, Cost-effective and rapid blood analysis on a cell-phone, *Lab Chip* 13, 2013, 1282–1288.
44. A. Coskun, J. Wong, D. Khodadadi, R Nagi, A Teya, A Ozcan, A personalized food allergen testing platform on a cellphone, *Lab Chip* 13, 2013, 636–640.
45. P. J. Hunt, E. A. Espiner, M. G. Nicholls, A. M. Richards, T. G. Yandle, The role of the circulation in processing pro- brain natriuretic peptide (proBNP) to amino-terminal BNP and BNP-32, *Peptides* 10, 1997, 1475–1481.
46. J. Goetze, J. Rehfeld, R. Videbaek, L. Friis-Hansen, J. Kastrup, B-type natriuretic peptide and its precursor in cardiac venous blood from failing hearts, *The European Journal of Heart Failure* 7, 2005, 69–74.
47. E. Reinhard, et al., *High Dynamic Range Imaging. Acquistion, Display, and Image-based Lightning*, Second Ed., Burlington MA: Morgan Kaufmann / Elsevier, 2010.
48. T. Chard, Pregnancy tests: A review, *Human Reproduction* 7, 1992, 701–710.
49. J. Penders, T. Fiers, J. Delanghe, Quantitative evaluation of urinalysis test strips, *Clinical Chemistry* 48, 2002, 2236–2241.
50. Test strips from EMD Millipore Brochure, EMD Millipore is a division of Merck KGaA, Darmstadt, Germany, http://www.merckmillipore.co.uk/chemicals/test-strips/c_Y_Ob.s1OpO0AAAEd1A41tk03? (26/03/14).
51. N. Oliver, C. Toumazou, A. Cass and D. Johnston, Glucose sensors: A review of current and emerging technology, *Diabet. Med.* 26, 2009, 197–210.
52. Cobas, Cobas h 232 POC-System, http://www.cobas.at/home/products_services/cobas_h_232_poc_system.html [in German]

53. D. Nagel, D. Seiler, E. Hohenberger, M. Ziegler, Investigations of ascorbic acid interference in urine test strips. *Clin. Lab.* 52, 2006, 149–153. https://www.poc.roche.com/poc/rewrite/generalContent/en_US/article/POC_general_article_70.htm, Urisys 1100 Operator's Manual, Roche Diagnostics, 2008.
54. A. Foudeh, T. Fatanat Didar, T. Veresa and M. Tabrizian, Microfluidic designs and techniques using lab-on-a-chip devices for pathogen detection for point-of-care diagnostics, *Lab Chip*, 2012, 12, 3249–3266.
55. P. Yager, T. Edwards, E. Fu, K. Helton, K. Nelson, M. Tam, B. Weigl, Microfluidic diagnostic technologies for global public health, *Nature* 442, 2006, 412–418.
56. B. Kuswandi, Nuriman, J. Huskens, W. Verboom, Optical sensing systems for microfluidic devices: A review, *Analytica Chimica Acta* 601, 2007, 141–155.
57. C. Chin, V. Linder, S. Sia, Lab-on-a-chip devices for global health: Past studies and future opportunities, *Lab Chip* 7, 2007, 41–57.
58. A. Martinez, S. Phillips, Z. Nie, C. Cheng, E. Carrilho, B. Wileya, G. Whitesides, Programmable diagnostic devices made from paper and tape, *Lab Chip* 10, 2010, 2499–2504.
59. W. Du, L. Li, K. Nichols, R. Ismagilov, SlipChip, *Lab Chip* 9, 2009, 2286–2292.
60. H. Liu, X. Li, R. Crooks, Paper-Based SlipPAD for High-Throughput Chemical Sensing, 2013, *in manuscript*.
61. H. Yu, G. Zhou, F. Chau, S. Sinh, Tunable electromagnetically actuated liquid-filled lens, *Sens. Actuat.* A 167, 2011, 602–607.
62. W. Zhang, K. Aljasem, H. Zappe, A. Seifert, Completely integrated, thermo-pneumatically tunable microlens, *Opt. Express* 19, 2011, 2347–2362.
63. C. Song, N. Nguyen, Y. Yap, T. Luong, A. Asundi, Multi-functional, optofluidic, in-plane, bi-concave lens: Tuning light beam from focused to divergent, *Microfluid. Nanofluid.* 10, 2011, 671–678.
64. P. Preechaburana, A. Suska, D. Filippini, Embedded adaptive optics for ubiquitous lab-on-a-chip readout on intact cell phones, *Sensors* 12, 2012, 8586–8600.
65. J. Homola, Surface plasmon resonance sensors for detection of chemical and biological species, *Chem. Rev.* 108, 2008, 462–493.
66. Biacore–GE, http://www.biacore.com (26/03/14).
67. Reichert Technologies, http://www.reichertspr.com (26/03/14).
68. Biosuplar, http://www.biosuplar.com (26/03/14).
69. Sensia, http://www.sensia.es/ (26/03/14).
70. M. Vala, K. Chadt, M. Piliarik, J. Homola, High-performance compact SPR sensor for multi-analyte sensing, *Sensors and Actuators* B 148, 2010, 544–549, and references therein.
71. Horiba Scientific, http://www.horiba.com/scientific/products/surface-plasmon-resonance-imaging-spri/ (26/03/14).
72. M. Chinowsky, J. Quinn, D. Bartholomew, R. Kaiser, J. Elkind, Performance of the Spreeta 2000 integrated surface plasmon resonance affinity sensor, *Sens. Actuators* B 69, 2003, 1–9.
73. Biacore 3000 Getting Started Kit, https://www.biacore.com/lifesciences/training/train_yourself/index.html?viewmode=printer (26/03/14).
74. B. Cunningham, J. Wang, I. Berggard, P. Peterson, Complete amino acid sequence of β_2-microglobulin, *Biochemistry* 12, 1974, 4811–4822.
75. M. Pignone, D. Nicoll, S. J. McPheke, *Pocket Guide to Diagnostic Tests*, New York: McGraw-Hill, 2004, p. 191.
76. R. Bharadwaj, A. Singh, Autonomous Lab-on-a-Chip Technologies, in *Autonomous Sensor Networks: Collective Sensing Strategies for Analytical Purposes*, D. Filippini (Ed.), Springer Series on Chemical Sensors and Biosensors (Series Ed. G. Urban), Volume 13, 2013, 217–236, Springer-Verlag, Berlin, Heidelberg.

77. I. K. Dimov, L. Basabe-Desmonts, J. L. Garcia-Cordero, B. M. Ross, A. J. Ricco, L. P. Lee, Stand-alone self-powered integrated microfluidic blood analysis system (SIMBAS), *Lab Chip* 11, 2011, 845–850.
78. J. Wang, H. Ahmad, C. Ma, Q. Shi, O. Vermesh, U. Vermesh, J. Heath, A self-powered, one-step chip for rapid, quantitative and multiplexed detection of proteins from pinpricks of whole blood, *Lab Chip* 10, 2010, 3157–3162.
79. P. Vulto, S. Podszun, P. Meyer, C. Hermann, A. Manzc, G. Urban, Phaseguides: A paradigm shift in microfluidic priming and emptying, *Lab Chip* 11, 2011, 1596–1602.
80. M. Zimmermann, P. Hunziker, E. Delamarche, Autonomous capillary system for one-step immunoassays, *Biomed Microdevices* 11, 2009, 1–8.
81. L. Gervais, E. Delamarche, Toward one-step point-of-care immunodiagnostics using capillary-driven microfluidics and PDMS substrates, *Lab Chip* 9, 2009, 3330–3337.
82. H. Chen, J. Cogswell, C. Anagnostopoulos, M. Faghri, A fluidic diode, valves, and a sequential-loading circuit fabricated on layered paper, *Lab Chip* 12, 2012, 2909–2913.

2 Lab on a Cellphone

Ahmet F. Coskun, Hongying Zhu, Onur Mudanyali, and Aydogan Ozcan

CONTENTS

2.1 INTRODUCTION

Today there are approximately 7 billion cellphone subscribers in the world, with a mobile phone penetration rate of ~96% globally [1]. In recent years, there has also been a significant increase in smartphone use especially in the developed parts of the world, which is projected to reach ~40% worldwide by 2015 [1]. Driven by this rapid growth of the mobile phone market, the cost of the cellphones has significantly decreased despite dramatic advances in the software and hardware components of these mobile technologies. To this end, the "state-of-art" digital components embedded in cellphones, including image sensors, micro-processors, displays, communication units etc., can be employed to create new opportunities for health monitoring in both the developed and the developing regions of the world. Therefore, cellphones, with their built-in features and global connectivity, can provide a ubiquitous platform for biomedical imaging, sensing, and diagnostics applications, which can potentially improve the health care delivery and help reduce the cost of biomedical tests worldwide by enabling the penetration of advanced microanalysis tools to even remote and resource-limited locations.

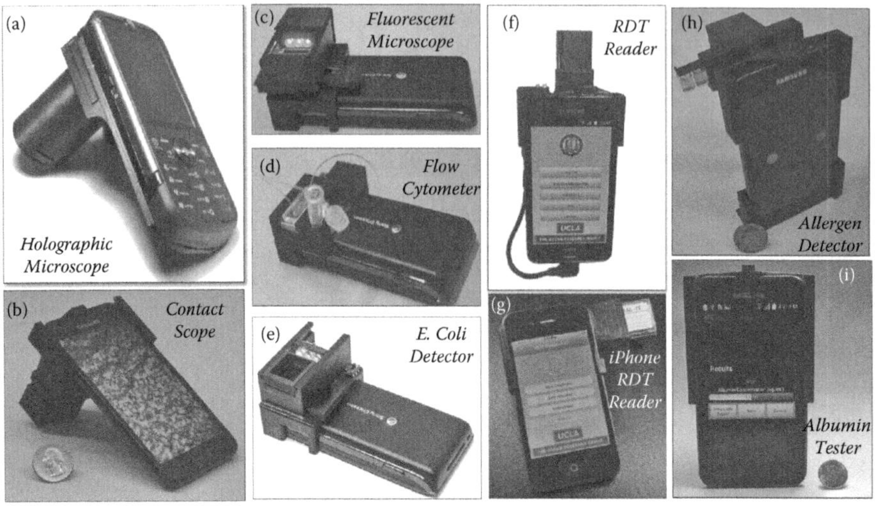

FIGURE 2.1 Mobile phone-based imaging and sensing technologies. (a) Lensfree holographic microscope, (b) multi-frame contact microscope, *Contact Scope*, (c) fluorescent microscope, (d) fluorescent imaging cytometer, (e) pathogen (e.g., *Escherichia Coli*) biosensor, (f–g) rapid diagnostic test reader, (h) food allergen (peanut) detector, (i) urinary albumin tester.

In this chapter, we review some of our group's recent efforts on developing *lab on a cellphone* platforms (see e.g., Figure 2.1) that aim to implement multiple telemedicine related functionalities on cellphones. Some of these emerging cellphone-based technologies that are detailed include: (1) transmission microscopes [2,3], (2) fluorescent microscopes and cytometers [4–6], (3) biosensors—particularly pathogen sensing systems [7], and (4) digital readers for rapid diagnostics tests [8–10]. In addition to their local use, we also present the spatio-temporal mapping of health related information and test results generated through these cellphone-based measurement and imaging technologies toward cloud-based health monitoring/tracking, also providing an important tool for epidemiology [11–13].

2.2 MOBILE IMAGING, SENSING, AND DIAGNOSTIC TECHNOLOGIES TOWARD LAB ON A CELLPHONE

Various biomedical tests are currently performed through the use of benchtop devices, where e.g., bodily fluids or biopsy samples collected from the patients are processed and analyzed using optical microscopes, flow-cytometers, plate or micro-well readers among others. These conventional biomedical tools, however, are relatively costly and rather bulky, making them less suitable for use in field or remote settings. In this section, we discuss some of the emerging mobile phone-based imaging and sensing tools that can perform microanalysis on various biological specimens through the use of transmission microscopy, fluorescent imaging and sensing, as well as digital read-outs for diagnostics tests.

2.2.1 Bright-Field Microscopy on a Cellphone

Optical microscopy has become one of the standard tools in biomedical sciences, especially for disease detection and diagnostics applications. In low-resource settings, for instance, bright-field microscopic evaluation of samples (e.g., sputum, tissue slices, as well as blood smears) remains as one of the primary methods for the diagnosis of infectious diseases, particularly for tuberculosis (TB) and malaria [14,15]. To create compact, lightweight, and cost-effective microscopic imaging tools, much research has been devoted to the development of mobile phone-based bright-field microscopes [2,3,16,17]. Although the specifications of these transmission microscopes vary based on their designs and working principles, a common feature is that an add-on opto-mechanical module is attached to the camera unit of a cellphone for image acquisition, which can then be processed on the same cellphone or transmitted to a central server/location for further processing, analysis, and reporting. Among these cellphone microscopes, we focus here on two computational methods that can be used to reduce the complexity of these imaging technologies while also enhancing the performance of the optical design: lensfree holographic imaging on a cellphone [2], and multi-frame contact imaging on a fiber-optic array using a smartphone [3] .

In the first computational imaging scheme, we demonstrated a lensfree digital microscopy platform on a cellphone as shown in Figure 2.1a [2]. This cellphone-based holographic microscope, weighing ~38 grams, does not use any lenses, lasers, or other bulky optical components, enabling a highly compact and lightweight imaging design that can be operated in field conditions. In this platform, we employ partially coherent illumination such as a simple light emitting diode (LED) that is filtered by a large pinhole (e.g., 0.1–0.2 mm) to illuminate the sample of interest, where the interference of the light waves passing through the micro-objects with the unperturbed background light creates the lensfree hologram of each micro-object, which is sampled/digitized at the CMOS (complementary metal-oxide semiconductor) detector array that is already embedded in the cellphone camera unit. These raw cellphone transmission images are then digitally processed through the use of a numerical method (based on, for example, phase retrieval algorithms) to compute the microscopic images of the samples of interest, yielding both the amplitude and phase information of the samples. Since we operate this imaging system under unit-fringe magnification, the imaging field of view (FOV) of this lensfree microscopy approach is equal to the active area of the sensor-array, typically achieving >20–30 mm^2 imaging area without the use of any mechanical scanners. We demonstrated the feasibility of this approach by imaging blood cells and waterborne parasites, among other microscopic objects. Such cellphone-based lensfree microscopes, together with their large FOV imaging capability, simplicity, and field-portability, hold promise for various telemedicine applications.

We also created a smartphone-based multi-frame contact imaging platform on a fiber-optic array [3], called *Contact Scope*, that can image highly dense or connected samples in transmission mode. This field-portable microscope (see Figure 2.2), weighing 76 grams, is also attached to the camera unit of a cellphone through the use of an add-on module, where planar samples of interest are positioned in contact with

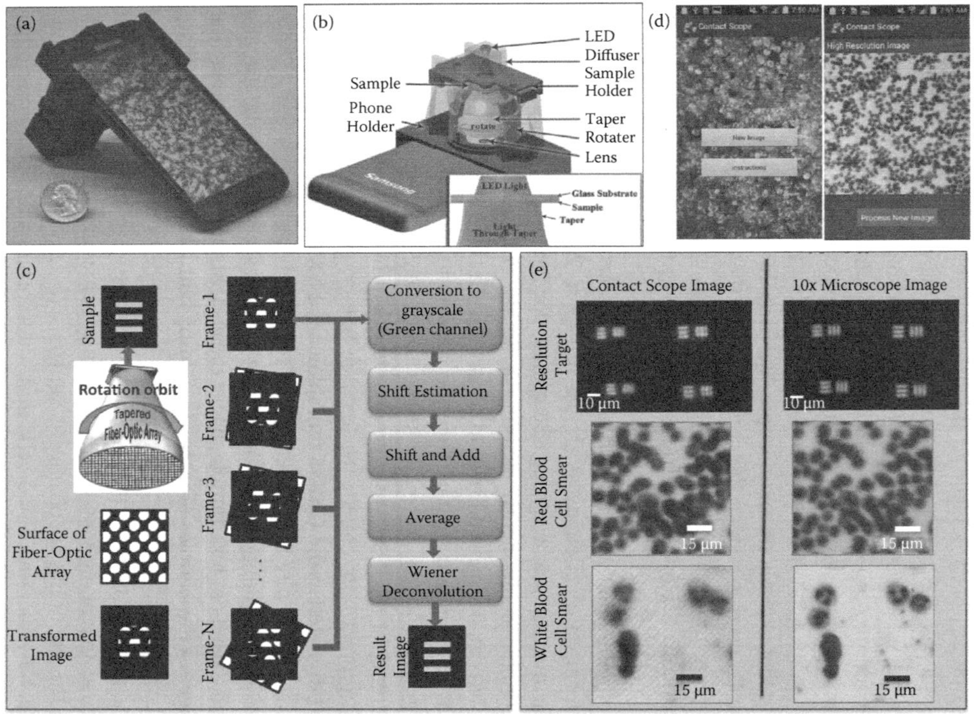

FIGURE 2.2 Smartphone-based multi-frame contact microscopy on a fiber-optic array, termed *Contact Scope*. (a) Photograph and (b) schematic of *Contact Scope*. (c) Working principle of multi-frame image acquisition and image reconstruction flow-chart. (d) Smart Android application running on the same cellphone for digital processing. (e) *Contact Scope*-based imaging of blood smears and corresponding 10X microscope image comparisons. (From Navruz, I. et al. 2013. "Smart-phone Based Computational Microscopy Using Multi-frame Contact Imaging on a Fiber-optic Array." *Lab on a Chip*, July 17. Reproduced by permission of The Royal Society of Chemistry.)

the top facet of a tapered fiber-optic array. Illuminating the sample using an incoherent light source such as a simple LED, this transmitted light pattern through the object is sampled by the fiber-optic array. After delivering this transmission image of the sample onto the other side of the taper with ~3X magnification in each direction, this magnified image of the object is projected onto the CMOS image sensor of the cellphone through the use of two lenses (one external lens in addition to the cellphone camera lens). Keeping the cellphone camera and the sample at a fixed position, the fiber-optic array is manually rotated with discrete angular increments of e.g., 1–2 degrees (see Figure 2.2c). Contact images are captured using the cellphone camera for each angular position of the taper, creating a sequence of transmission images of the same sample. These multi-frame images are then digitally combined based on a shift-and-add algorithm through a custom-developed Android application running on the smartphone (see Figure 2.2d), yielding the final microscopic image of the sample, which can also be accessed through the cellphone screen.

We reported the performance of this *Contact Scope* platform by imaging resolution test charts and blood smears as shown in Figure 2.2e, demonstrating that this platform can achieve >1.5–2.5 μm spatial resolution over a FOV of e.g., >1.5–15 mm^2. This cellphone-based computational contact microscopy platform, being compact and lightweight, also employing rapid digital processing running on smartphones, could be useful for point-of-care applications.

2.2.2 Fluorescent Microscopy and Cytometry on a Cellphone

In addition to the bright-field imaging modalities implemented on cellphones, other optical microscopy techniques including e.g., dark-field microscopy and fluorescence microscopy can also be integrated with cellphones for telemedicine applications. Fluorescent microscopy deserves special attention as it might enhance the sensitivity and specificity in e.g., image-based disease detection and diagnosis. Therefore, combining fluorescent microscopy with cellphone technologies might be rather useful for field-diagnostics needs.

Toward this end, our lab has developed a compact and cost-effective cellphone-based fluorescent microscope [5] that can image and analyze fluorescently labeled specimens without the use of any bulky optical components. As shown in Figure 2.1c,d, the major components of this cost-effective platform include a simple lens, a plastic color filter, LEDs, and batteries. In this platform, the excitation light generated by e.g., LEDs illuminates the sample from the side using lensfree butt coupling to the sample cuvette. Due to the large cross-section of the LED light, this coupling is quite insensitive to alignment, which makes it repeatable from sample to sample. In this design, the sample holder microchip (where the liquid specimen is located) can be considered to be a multi-mode slab waveguide, which has a layered refractive index structure. Such a multi-layered slab waveguide has strong refractive index contrast at the air-glass (or polydimethylsiloxane [PDMS]) interfaces (i.e., the top and the bottom surfaces), as a result of which the pump/excitation photons are tightly guided within this waveguide. On the other hand, the refractive index contrast at glass (or PDMS)-sample solution interfaces is much weaker compared to air-glass interfaces, which permit a significant portion of the pump photons to leak into the sample solution to efficiently excite e.g., labeled bacteria/pathogens suspended within the liquid sample. Together with this guided-wave-based excitation of specimen located within a microchip, the fluorescent emission from the labeled targets is collected by a simple lens system to be imaged onto the cellphone CMOS sensor. For this fluorescent imaging geometry, the image magnification is determined by f/f_2, where f is focal length of the cellphone camera (e.g., $f \sim 4.65$ mm for the cellphone model: Sony-Erickson U10i) and f_2 is the focal length of the add-on lens. Depending on the application and its requirements on resolution and FOV, different magnification factors can be achieved by varying f_2 value. Note also that this magnification factor is theoretically independent of the distance between the two lenses, which makes alignment of our attachment to the cellphone rather easy and repeatable.

This imaging configuration, when the fluorescent objects are imaged in static mode, is used as a fluorescent microscope as shown in Figure 2.1c. When the fluorescent objects are flowing through the microfluidic channel and their images are recorded in the video mode, the device can be used as a fluorescent imaging cytometer [4] to count the fluorescent objects flowing through the microfluidic chamber as illustrated in Figure 2.1d. This scheme can also be used to count cell densities, such as the density of white blood cells in whole blood samples as demonstrated in e.g. [4].

Quite recently, we have also changed the design of this cellphone-based fluorescent microscopy platform to detect individual virus particles [18]. In this imaging design, a miniature laser diode is used to excite the fluorescently labeled virus particles with an highly oblique illumination angle (e.g. ~75°), which helps us create a decent dark-field background since the low numerical aperture of the cellphone imaging optics misses most of these oblique excitation photons, enhancing our contrast and signal-to-noise ratio so that individual viruses and deeply sub-wavelength fluorescent particles (e.g., 90–100 nm in diameter) can be detected on the cellphone. This single nanoparticle detection and counting capability can especially be important for viral load measurements in field conditions.

2.2.3 Biosensing on a Cellphone

Together with the recent progress in the development of fluorescent imaging modalities on cellphones, we also expanded this cellphone-based fluorescent detection geometry to various biosensing applications, including for example the detection of pathogens (e.g., *Escherichia coli*) toward screening of liquid samples such as water and milk [7]). In this scheme (see Figure 2.3), we utilized antibody functionalized glass capillaries as solid substrates to perform quantum dot-based sandwich assay for specific and sensitive detection of *E. coli* in liquid samples of interest (see Figure 2.3b). The *E. coli* particles captured on the inner surfaces of these functionalized capillaries are then excited using inexpensive LEDs, where we image the fluorescent emission from the quantum dots using the cellphone's CMOS sensor utilizing an additional lens that is placed in front of the camera unit of the phone. We then quantify the *E. coli* concentration in liquid samples by integrating the fluorescent signal per capillary tube.

We validated the performance of this cellphone-based *E. coli* detection platform in buffer and fat-free milk samples (see Figure 2.3c,d), achieving a detection limit of

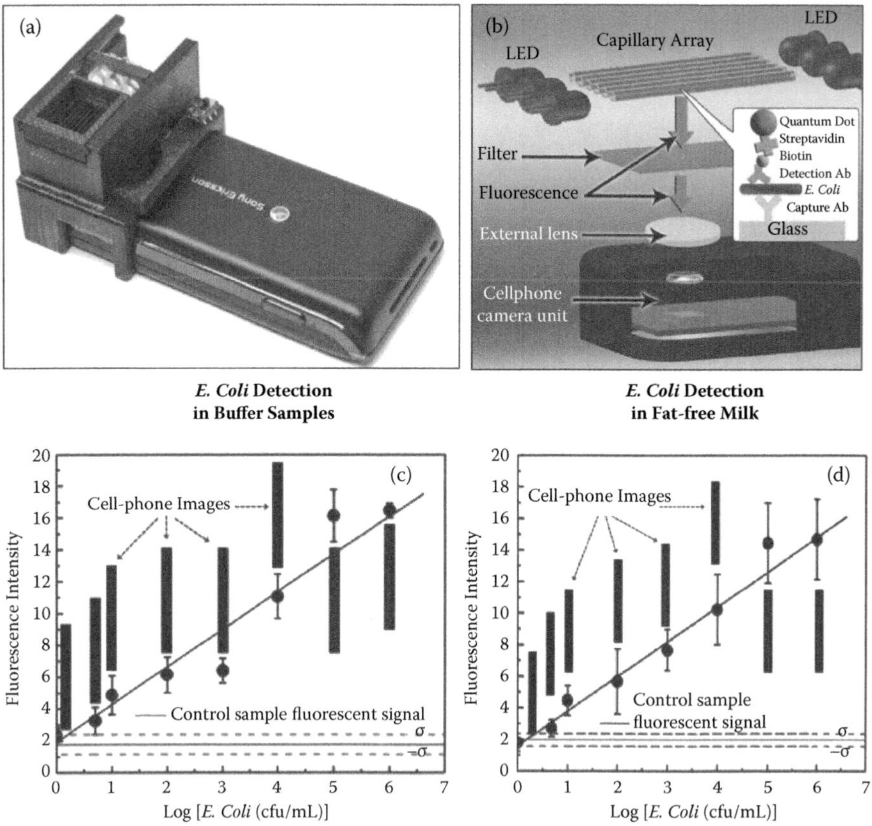

FIGURE 2.3 Detection of *E. coli* on a cellphone. (a) Picture and (b) schematic of the cellphone-based *E. Coli* detector. (c) Validation of *E. Coli* detection in buffer samples and (d) in fat-free milk specimen. (From Zhu, H., U. Sikora, and A. Ozcan. 2012. "Quantum Dot Enabled Detection of *Escherichia Coli* Using a Cell-phone." *Analyst* 137, 11, May 7: 2541–2544. Reproduced by permission of The Royal Society of Chemistry.)

~5–10 cfu per mL in both specimens. Such a pathogen detection platform installed on cellphones, being field-portable and cost-effective, could be useful for e.g., rapid screening of water and food samples in low resource settings.

2.2.4 Blood Analysis on a Cellphone

One of the important applications of cellphone-based imaging and sensing is to perform rapid and cost-effective blood analysis. Toward this need, as shown in Figure 2.4, an automated blood analysis platform running on a smartphone [6] has been created which consists of two parts: (1) a base attachment to the cellphone that includes batteries and a universal port for three different add-on attachments; and (2) opto-mechanical add-on components for white blood cell and red blood cell counting as well as hemoglobin density measurements. Each one of these attachments has

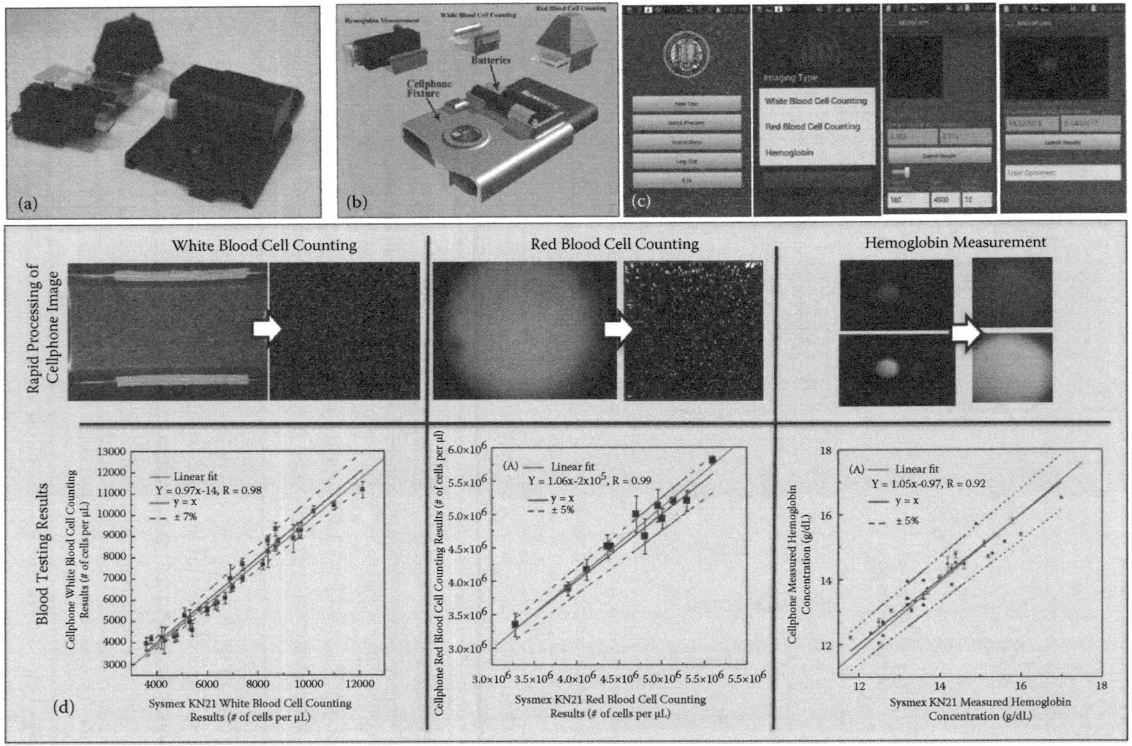

FIGURE 2.4 Rapid and cost-effective blood analysis on a smartphone. (a) Photograph and (b) schematic of the cellphone-based blood analyzer. (c) Android application running on the same smart phone for automated digital processing and quantification. (d) Blood testing results with the white blood cell counts, red blood cell counts, and hemoglobin concentration measurements. (From Zhu, H. et al. 2013. "Cost-effective and Rapid Blood Analysis on a Cell-phone." *Lab on a Chip* 13, 7, March 5: 1282–1288. Reproduced by permission of The Royal Society of Chemistry.)

a plano-convex lens and an LED source. When a specific attachment is clicked onto the cellphone base, the plano-convex lens in that component gets in contact with the existing lens of the cellphone camera, creating a microscopic imaging geometry that forms the images of the biological specimen (e.g., blood cells) located within disposable sample holders on the cellphone sensor-array. For blood analysis, white blood cells are fluorescently labeled and imaged using an opto-fluidic illumination scheme as described earlier [5]. Unlabeled intact red blood cells are imaged using a bright-field illumination mode, and hemoglobin concentration is estimated based on the measurement of absorbance of the lysed blood sample [6]. A custom-designed Android application is also created to directly process the obtained images on the cellphone (see Figure 2.4). This Android application reports the test results in terms of "number of cells per microliter" and "gram per deciliter" for blood cell counts and hemoglobin concentration measurements, respectively.

We tested the blood samples from anonymous donors to evaluate the performance of this cellphone-based blood analyzer (see Figure 2.4d). For white blood cells (WBCs), we typically counted 600 to 2500 cells per fluorescent image within a FOV of ~ 21 mm^2. The absolute error is within 7% of the standard test results obtained using a commercially available blood analyzer [6]. For red blood cells (RBCs), we counted around 400 to 700 cells per image within a FOV of 1.2 mm^2. The absolute error for RBC tests is within 5% of the standard test results. For hemoglobin tests, we first measured the transmission intensity of water samples over a FOV of ~9 mm^2, followed by the measurement of the transmission light intensity of lysed blood samples over the same FOV. We calculated the blood sample absorbance based on these differential measurements. This measured sample absorbance value was then compared to a calibration curve obtained for our platform and hemoglobin concentration in the unknown sample was estimated based on this linear fitting. This process generated an absolute hemoglobin density measurement error within 5% of the standard test results obtained using a commercially available blood analyzer.

2.2.5 Integrated Rapid-Diagnostic-Test Reader on a Cellphone

Cellphone-based imaging technologies can also be employed as digital readers for diagnostics tests used especially in developing parts of the world. Since monitoring public health threats is a challenging task in remote locations due to the lack of trained health care personnel and advanced medical instrumentation, the use of rapid diagnostic tests (RDTs), e.g., lateral flow-based chromatographic assays, offers significant advantages, superseding clinical examination and other traditional approaches. Special biomarkers in bodily fluids (e.g., saliva, urine, and blood) during an infection or medical condition develop color changes on chromatographic RDTs that are conventionally read via visual inspection by the human eye. However, quantitative and multiplexed chromatographic RDTs have been emerging as part of the next generation diagnostics tools, enabling highly sensitive and accurate diagnostics beyond the limited functions of qualitative RDTs [19–22].

To provide a compact and cost-effective solution to this important task of quantitative reading of diagnostics tests, cellphones can be utilized to digitize, interpret, store, and transfer the information acquired using these state-of-art multiplexed

RDTs. Toward this direction, we demonstrated a cellphone- based "universal" RDT reader platform (see Figure 2.5a) that enables digital evaluation of various types of chromatographic RDTs using a lightweight and cost-effective snap-on attachment (see Figure 2.5b) together with a custom-developed cellphone application (for both iPhone and Android operating systems) as shown in Figure 2.5c [8]. Weighing ~65 grams, this cellphone attachment comprises an inexpensive plano-convex lens and multiple diffused light-emitting diode (LED) arrays powered by the cellphone battery through a USB (universal serial bus) cable or two AAA batteries (see Figure 2.5b). This opto-mechanical unit can be repeatedly attached to and detached from the back of the existing cellphone camera to digitally acquire the images of RDTs in reflection or transmission modes which are processed in real time using the cellphone application to generate a test report including the patient information, test validation, test result, and the quantification of the test signal intensities. The same cellphone application can then store these test reports locally on the cellphone or wirelessly transmit them to a secure database to generate a real-time spatio-temporal map of test results and other conditions (e.g., anthrax attacks or aflatoxin contamination) that can be diagnosed or sensed using RDTs (see Figure 2.6) [8].

Performance of this integrated platform has been demonstrated by imaging various different chromatographic RDTs including Optimal-IT Malaria Tests (Bio-Rad Laboratories, California), HIV 1/2 Ab PLUS Combo Rapid Tests as well as TB IgG/IgM Combo Rapid Tests (CTK Biotech, California) [23–26]. RDTs activated with whole blood samples and positive control wells were successfully imaged using this cellphone-based smart RDT reader to validate the accuracy and repeatability of our measurements (see Figure 2.5d).

In order to demonstrate the sensitivity of our platform, we also imaged Optimal-IT Malaria RDTs that were activated using various different concentration levels of antigens. Starting with the manufacturer recommended dilution level of Positive Control Well Antigen (PCWA)/20 μl (1x dilution), we diluted the antigens by 2, 3, and 4 times to create concentration levels of PCWA/40 μl (2x dilution), PCWA/60 μl (3x dilution), and PCWA/80 μl (4x dilution), respectively, and activated 10 RDTs for each concentration level. Our digital reader imaged and correctly evaluated all the RDTs that were activated with PCWA/20 μl, PCWA/40 μl as well as PCWA/60 μl, providing "valid and positive" in the final test reports. On the other hand, due to the weak signal intensity on the RDTs activated with PCWA/80 μl, i.e., at 4x dilution compared to the recommended level, the accuracy of our reader dropped to ~60% (see Figure 2.5e).

This cellphone-based RDT reader platform enables digital and quantitative evaluation of various RDTs that are taking the center stage of point-of-care diagnostics in remote locations. Generating a real-time spatio-temporal map of epidemics and other public health threats that can be diagnosed using RDTs, this integrated platform can be useful for policy makers, health care specialists, and epidemiologists to monitor the occurrence and spread of various conditions and might assist us to react in a timely manner.

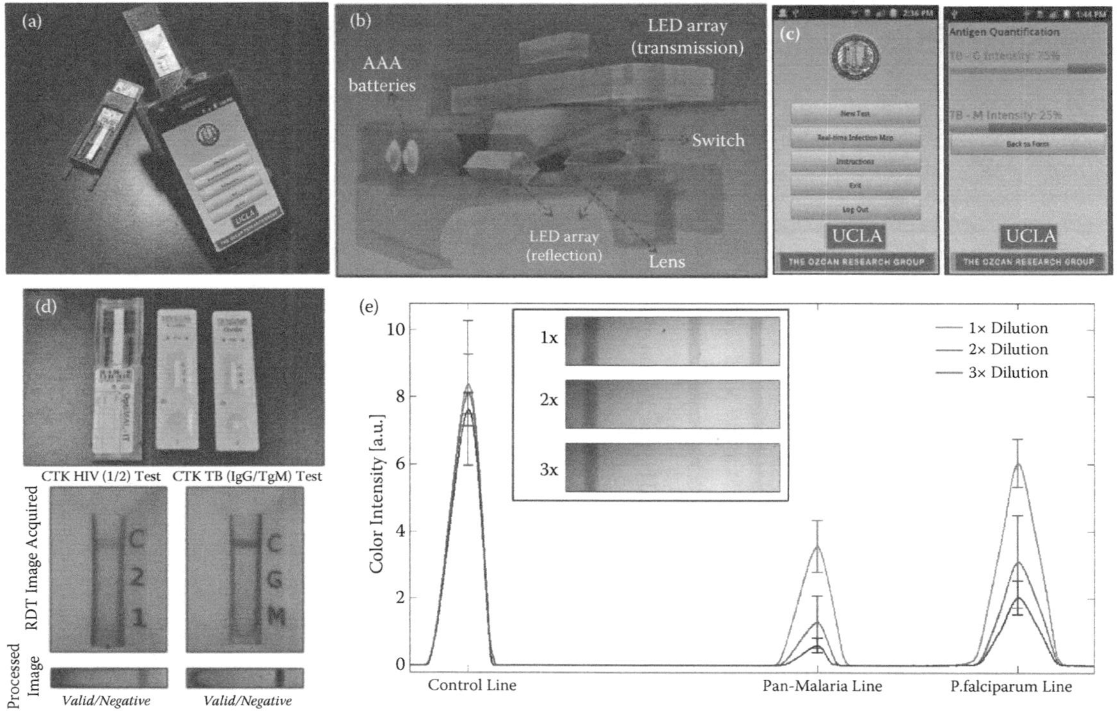

FIGURE 2.5 Integrated rapid diagnostic test reader on a cellphone. (a) Picture and (b) schematic of the cellphone-based RDT reader platform. (c) Custom developed application running on the same Android phone for digital antigen quantification and validation. (d) Various RDTs (HIV and TB) with their corresponding raw and processed cellphone images. (e) Smartphone-based quantification of malaria RDTs activated using various different concentration levels of antigens. (From Mudanyali, O. et al. 2012. "Integrated Rapid-Diagnostic-Test Reader Platform on a Cellphone." *Lab on a Chip* 12, 15, August 7: 2678–2686. Reproduced by permission of The Royal Society of Chemistry.)

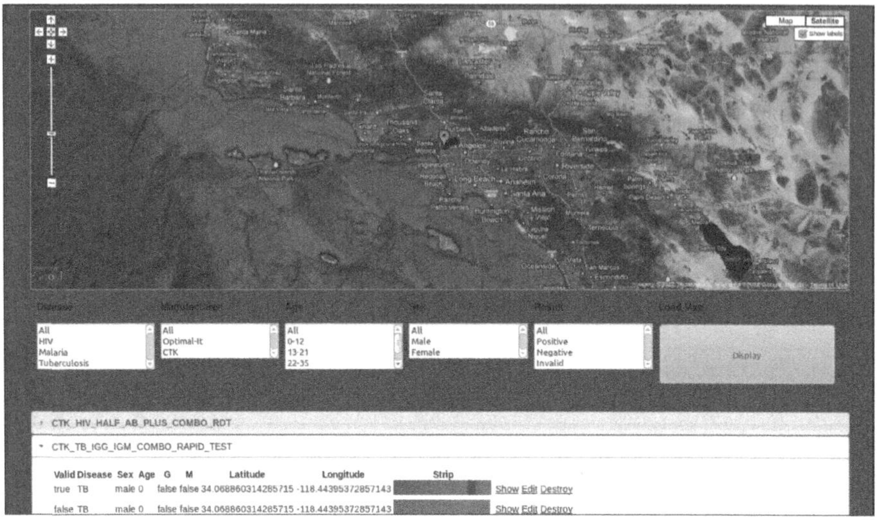

FIGURE 2.6 Spatio-temporal mapping of infectious diseases. Cellphone-based RDT-reader generated test reports and patient data uploaded to a central database. (From Mudanyali, O. et al. 2012. "Integrated Rapid-Diagnostic-Test Reader Platform on a Cellphone." *Lab on a Chip* 12, 15, August 7: 2678–2686. Reproduced by permission of The Royal Society of Chemistry.)

2.2.6 Albumin Testing in Urine Using a Cellphone

Some of these emerging mobile phone-based diagnostics platforms can also be utilized for monitoring chronic patients. As an example, chronic kidney disease patients or other patients who suffer from diabetes, hypertension, and/or cardiovascular diseases, might potentially benefit from health screening applications running on cellphones, enabling frequent and routine testing in public settings including e.g., homes, offices, etc. Along these lines, we have recently developed a personalized digital sensing platform, termed *Albumin Tester*, running on a smartphone [10] that images and automatically analyzes fluorescent assays enclosed within disposable test tubes toward specific and sensitive detection of albumin in urine. Using a mechanical attachment mounted on the camera unit of a cellphone (see Figure 2.7a,b), test and control tubes are excited by a battery powered laser diode, where the laser beam interacts with the control tube after probing the sample of interest located within the test tube. We capture the images of fluorescent tubes using the cellphone camera through the use of an external lens that is inserted between the sample and the camera lens. These fluorescent images of the sample and control tubes are then digitally processed within 1 second through the use of an Android application (see Figure 2.7c) running on the same phone, providing the quantification of albumin concentration in the urine specimen of interest.

To validate the performance of this cellphone-based *Albumin Tester*, we tested buffer samples spiked with albumin proteins at various concentrations covering 0 μg/mL, 10 μg/mL, 25 μg/mL, 50 μg/mL, 100 μg/mL, 200 μg/mL, 250 μg/mL, and 300 μg/mL. Based on three different measurements for each concentration, we

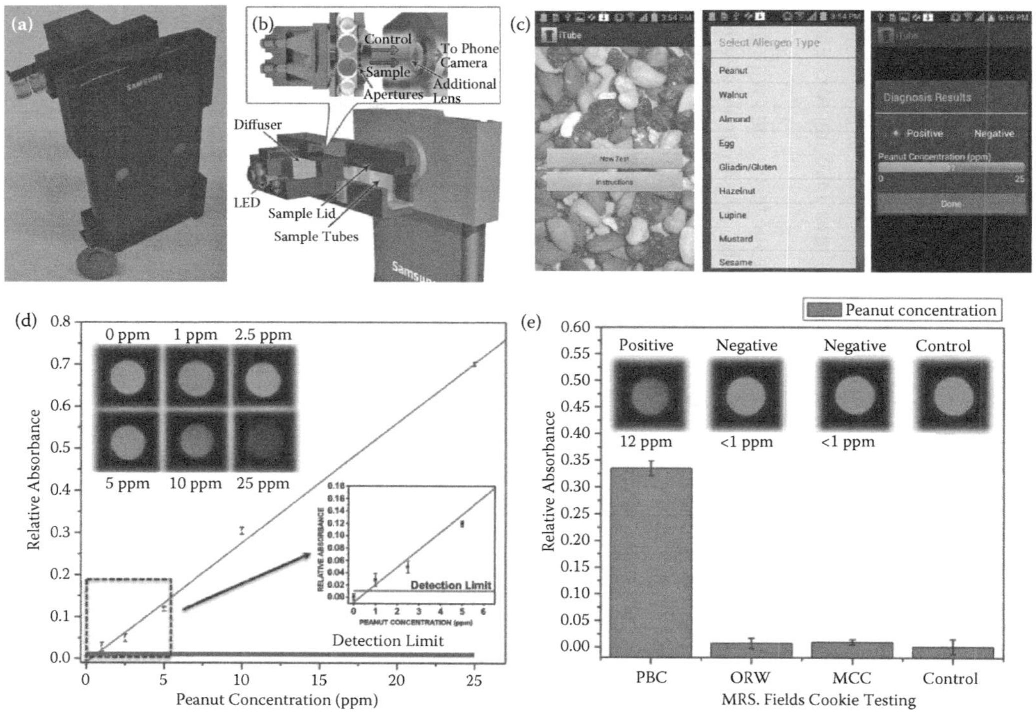

FIGURE 2.7 Allergen testing on a smartphone. (a) Picture and (b) schematic diagram of *iTube*. (c) Custom Android application for allergen quantification on the same smartphone. (d) Calibration of *iTube* based on the experiments performed with samples containing known concentrations of peanut. (e) Testing of commercially available cookies through the use of *iTube*. (From Coskun, A. et al. 2013. "A Personalized Food Allergen Testing Platform on a Cellphone." *Lab on a Chip* 13, 4, January 24: 636–640. Reproduced by permission of The Royal Society of Chemistry.)

obtained a dose-response curve (see Figure 2.7d) that demonstrates the linear relationship between the spiked albumin concentration in buffer and corresponding relative fluorescent unit (RFU = $I_{test}/I_{control}$, where I_{test} and $I_{control}$ are the *fluorescent* signal of the sample tube and the control tube, respectively) values, achieving a detection limit of ~5–10 μg/mL in buffer. Next, we performed measurements in synthetic urine samples (see Figure 2.7d) spiked with albumin proteins at different concentrations spanning 0 μg/mL, 10 μg/mL, 25 μg/mL, 50 μg/mL, 100 μg/mL, and 200 μg/mL. Similar to our buffer experiments, these experiments achieved an albumin detection limit of <10 μg/mL in urine samples. Furthermore, we also performed blind experiments (see Figure 2.7e) with albumin spiked synthetic urine samples at randomly selected concentrations (i.e., 200, 150, 25, 10, 100, and 50 μg/mL), where the albumin concentration of each unknown urine sample is estimated with an absolute error of <7 μg/mL based on the calibration curve presented in Figure 2.7d. For these measurements, sample preparation and incubation procedures take approximately 5 minutes per test.

The users of this *Albumin Tester* platform can also share the test results with their doctors by uploading the data to secure central servers. Such a personalized albumin testing tool running on smartphones, with its sensitivity level that is more than 3 times lower than clinically accepted normal range for urinary albumin concentration (~30 μg/mL), could impact early diagnosis of kidney disease or remote monitoring of chronic patients.

2.2.7 Food Allergen Testing on a Cellphone

In parallel to the utilization of cellphone-based imaging and sensing platforms for the diagnosis or monitoring of diseases, another important public concern that could benefit from cellphone-based testing platforms is the detection of allergens in food samples. To this end, we devised a personalized food allergen testing platform [9], termed *iTube*, running on a smartphone that images and automatically analyzes colorimetric assays performed in test tubes for specific and sensitive detection of allergens in food products (see Figure 2.8). Utilizing a compact mechanical attachment installed on the camera unit of a cellphone (see Figure 2.8a,b), we capture the transmission images of our test and control tubes under vertical illumination by two separate LEDs. In this process, allergen assay within the tubes absorbs the illumination light which changes the intensity in the acquired cellphone image. Digitally processing these transmission images of the sample and control tubes within 1 second through the use of a custom-developed Android application (see Figure 2.8c), the same smartphone application provides the test results, quantifying the allergen contamination in food products.

To demonstrate its proof of concept, we used our *iTube* platform for specific testing of peanut concentration in food products. Initially, we calibrated our *iTube* platform (see Figure 2.8d) by measuring known amounts of peanut concentration spanning 0 ppm, 1 ppm, 2.5 ppm, 5 ppm, 10 ppm, and 25 ppm based on a sample preparation and incubation time of ~20 min per test. Digitally quantifying these samples through the use of the *iTube* platform, we determined the relative absorbance, defined as $A = \log_{10} (I_{control}/I_{test}$, where $I_{control}$ and I_{test} are the total *transmitted*

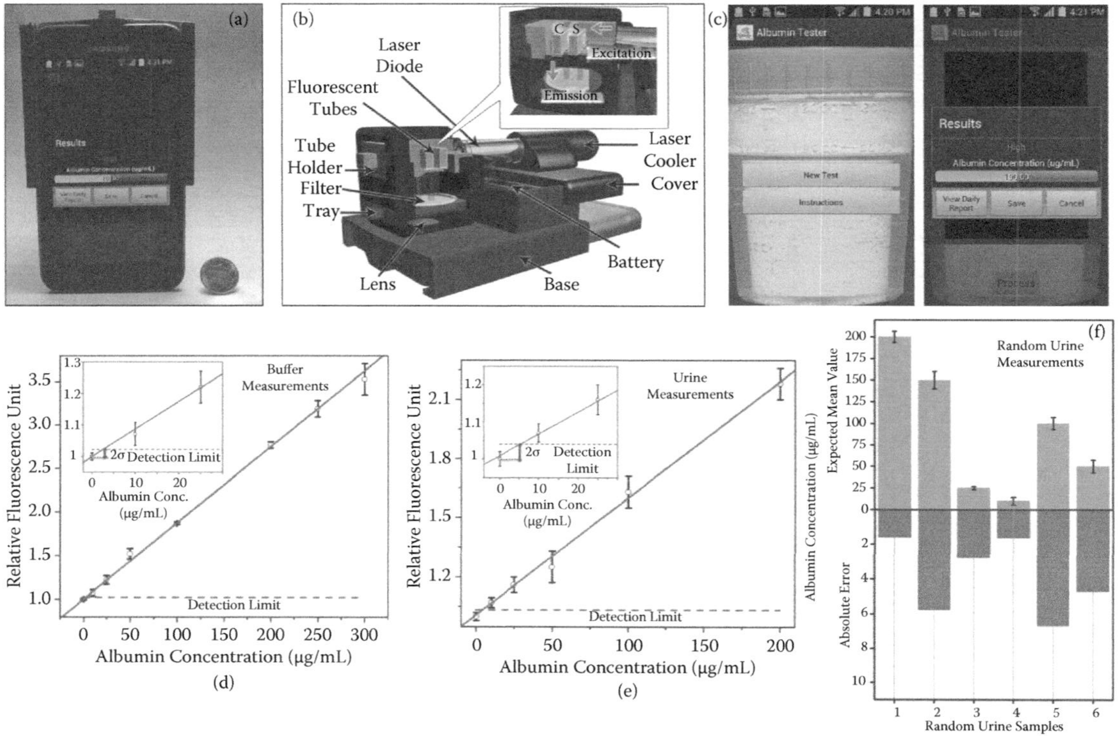

FIGURE 2.8 Urinary albumin testing on a smart phone, termed as *Albumin Tester*. (a) Photograph and (b) schematic of *Albumin Tester*. (c) An Android application installed on the same smartphone for quantification of albumin concentration in the urine sample of interest. Calibration of *Albumin Tester* based on the measurements performed in (d) buffer samples and in (e) synthetic urine specimen, both of which were spiked with albumin proteins at various concentrations. (f) Urinary albumin testing in randomly selected samples through the *Albumin Tester*. (From Coskun, A. et al. 2013. "Albumin Testing in Urine Using a Smart-phone." *Lab on a Chip*, 13, 4231–4238 (2013). Reproduced by permission of The Royal Society of Chemistry.)

signal through the control tube and the sample tube, respectively), of each test tube, yielding a calibration curve that can be used to quantify the allergen concentration (C) in any given food product of interest based on the measured relative absorbance value (i.e., A) of the target sample.

Next, we tested three different kinds of commercially available cookies for their peanut concentrations and quantified the level of peanut in these products based on the calibration curve presented in Figure 2.8d. As summarized in Figure 2.8e, our *iTube* platform achieved the following results: (i) peanut butter chocolate (PBC) cookie was found to be positive (as expected) with an absorbance value of 0.33, equivalent to a peanut concentration of 12 ppm. Since we diluted this PBC extract approximately 5,000 times using phosphate buffered saline (PBS) solution to avoid signal saturation, the real peanut concentration of this PBS sample was more than 60,000 ppm. This large dilution, however, is not required for practical uses as our *iTube* platform aims to detect "hidden" allergen cross-contamination in food products and therefore saturation of our measurement reading is not a practical issue or concern. (ii) Oatmeal raisin with walnut (ORW) cookie was found to be negative with negligible absorbance, equivalent to a peanut concentration of less than 1 ppm, which implies that walnut existence in this sample did not interfere with our testing results. (iii) Milk chocolate chip (MCC) cookie was also found to be negative with negligible absorbance, equivalent to peanut concentration of less than 1 ppm.

Allergic individuals using our *iTube* platform can upload their test results to a central server to create a personalized or public (if desired) testing archive. The spatio-temporal analysis of this allergy database might also impact food related regulations and policies.

2.3 DISCUSSION AND CONCLUSIONS

In this chapter, we presented digital imaging, sensing, and diagnostics platforms running on cellphones that can provide various solutions for existing public health needs and global health problems through microanalysis performed on bodily fluids (e.g., urine, blood), screening of pathogens in liquid samples, or detection of allergens in food samples. In addition to the approaches discussed earlier, several other recent works also provided innovative uses of cellphone-based technologies in biomedical applications, including label-free spectroscopic biosensors [27], electrochemical biosensors [28], pH sensors [29,30], surface plasmon resonance chemical sensors [31], and lab-on-a-card readers [32], among others. All these complementary efforts, aiming to build a multi-functional portable laboratory integrated onto cellphones, might improve access to affordable and personalized health care through state-of-art digital imaging, sensing, and diagnostics components and smart applications running on cellphones.

Furthermore, these cellphone-based microanalysis and diagnostics tools, with their connectivity worldwide, can be digitally linked to each other and to central servers, where massive amounts of biomedical data can be securely (although the security and encryption of almost any data can be broken at the cost of computation time) shared and stored in cloud-based networks to create spatio-temporal databases or maps for e.g., various diseases, hazardous biomarkers, pathogenic organisms, and many others. This cloud-based smart global health system might be valuable for telemedicine applications, epidemics, and endemics research, providing a much needed epidemiology tool.

Finally, we should also note that the rapid evolution of cellphone hardware and software as well as configuration differences from wireless carrier to carrier pose limitations for dissemination and potential commercialization of some of the above described cellphone-based sensing and imaging technologies. To address this challenge, second-hand or refurbished cellphones can be utilized for the development of these cellphone-based telemedicine platforms as an alternative business strategy, providing device designers and diagnostics companies with a supply of reliable, inexpensive, relatively older-generation phones which can potentially assist the growth and sustainability of the mobile health care market, especially in the developing world, where the smartphone penetration is still at its infancy and the cost of the final product is very sensitive.

Conflicts of Interest Statement: A.O. is the cofounder of a startup company (Holomic LLC) which aims to commercialize computational imaging and sensing technologies licensed from UCLA.

ACKNOWLEDGMENTS

Ozcan Research Group gratefully acknowledges the support of the Presidential Early Career Award for Scientists and Engineers (PECASE), Army Research Office (ARO) Life Sciences Division, ARO Young Investigator Award, National Science Foundation (NSF) CAREER Award, NSF CBET Biophotonics Program, NSF EFRI Award, Office of Naval Research (ONR) Young Investigator Award, and National Institutes of Health (NIH) Director's New Innovator Award DP2OD006427 from the Office of the Director, National Institutes of Health.

REFERENCES

1. "The World in 2013: ICT Facts and Figures." 2013. *ITU*. Accessed July 27. http://www.itu.int/en/ITU-D/Statistics/Pages/facts/default.aspx.
2. Tseng, Derek, Onur Mudanyali, Cetin Oztoprak, Serhan O. Isikman, Ikbal Sencan, Oguzhan Yaglidere, and Aydogan Ozcan. 2010. "Lensfree Microscopy on a Cellphone." *Lab on a Chip* 10(14) (June 29):1787–1792. doi:10.1039/C003477K.
3. Navruz, Isa, Ahmet F. Coskun, Justin Wong, Saqib Mohammad, Derek Tseng, Richie Nagi, Stephen Phillips, and Aydogan Ozcan. 2013. "Smart-phone Based Computational Microscopy Using Multi-frame Contact Imaging on a Fiber-optic Array." *Lab on a Chip* 13(20) (Oct. 21), 4015–4023, 2013.
4. Zhu, Hongying, Sam Mavandadi, Ahmet F. Coskun, Oguzhan Yaglidere, and Aydogan Ozcan. 2011. "Optofluidic Fluorescent Imaging Cytometry on a Cell Phone." *Analytical Chemistry* 83(17) (September 1):6641–6647. doi:10.1021/ac201587a.
5. Zhu, Hongying, Oguzhan Yaglidere, Ting-Wei Su, Derek Tseng, and Aydogan Ozcan. 2011. "Cost-effective and Compact Wide-field Fluorescent Imaging on a Cell-phone." *Lab on a Chip* 11(2) (January 21):315–322. doi:10.1039/C0LC00358A.

6. Zhu, Hongying, Ikbal Sencan, Justin Wong, Stoyan Dimitrov, Derek Tseng, Keita Nagashima, and Aydogan Ozcan. 2013. "Cost-effective and Rapid Blood Analysis on a Cell-phone." *Lab on a Chip* 13(7) (March 5):1282–1288. doi:10.1039/C3LC41408F.
7. Zhu, Hongying, Uzair Sikora, and Aydogan Ozcan. 2012. "Quantum Dot Enabled Detection of *Escherichia Coli* Using a Cell-phone." *Analyst* 137(11) (May 7):2541–2544. doi:10.1039/C2AN35071H.
8. Mudanyali, Onur, Stoyan Dimitrov, Uzair Sikora, Swati Padmanabhan, Isa Navruz, and Aydogan Ozcan. 2012. "Integrated Rapid-Diagnostic-Test Reader Platform on a Cellphone." *Lab on a Chip* 2012,12, 2678–2686.
9. Coskun, Ahmet F., Justin Wong, Delaram Khodadadi, Richie Nagi, Andrew Tey, and Aydogan Ozcan. 2013. "A Personalized Food Allergen Testing Platform on a Cellphone." *Lab on a Chip* 13(4) (January 24):636–640. doi:10.1039/C2LC41152K.
10. Coskun, Ahmet F., Richie Nagi, Kayvon Sadeghi, Stephen Phillips, and Aydogan Ozcan. 2013. "Albumin Testing in Urine Using a Smart-phone." *Lab on a Chip*, 13, 4231–4238 (2013).
11. Mavandadi, Sam, Stoyan Dimitrov, Steve Feng, Frank Yu, Uzair Sikora, Oguzhan Yaglidere, Swati Padmanabhan, Karin Nielsen, and Aydogan Ozcan. 2012. "Distributed Medical Image Analysis and Diagnosis through Crowd-Sourced Games: A Malaria Case Study." *PLoS ONE* 7(5) (May 11):e37245. doi:10.1371/journal.pone.0037245.
12. Mavandadi, Sam, Stoyan Dimitrov, Steve Feng, Frank Yu, Richard Yu, Uzair Sikora, and Aydogan Ozcan. 2012. "Crowd-sourced BioGames: Managing the Big Data Problem for Next-Generation Lab-on-a-Chip Platforms." *Lab on a Chip* 12(20) (September 18):4102–4106. doi:10.1039/C2LC40614D.
13. Mavandadi, Sam, Steve Feng, Frank Yu, Stoyan Dimitrov, Richard Yu, and Aydogan Ozcan. 2012. "BioGames: A Platform for Crowd-Sourced Biomedical Image Analysis and Telediagnosis." *Games for Health Journal* 1(5) (October):373–376. doi:10.1089/g4h.2012.0054.
14. Makler, M.T., C.J. Palmer, and A.L. Ager. 1998. "A Review of Practical Techniques for the Diagnosis of Malaria." *Annals of Tropical Medicine and Parasitology* 92(4) (June):419–433.
15. Steingart, Karen R., Vivienne Ng, Megan Henry, Philip C. Hopewell, Andrew Ramsay, Jane Cunningham, Richard Urbanczik, Mark D. Perkins, Mohamed Abdel Aziz, and Madhukar Pai. 2006. "Sputum Processing Methods to Improve the Sensitivity of Smear Microscopy for Tuberculosis: A Systematic Review." *The Lancet Infectious Diseases* 6(10) (October):664–674. doi:10.1016/S1473-3099(06)70602-8.
16. Breslauer, David N., Robi N. Maamari, Neil A. Switz, Wilbur A. Lam, and Daniel A. Fletcher. 2009. "Mobile Phone Based Clinical Microscopy for Global Health Applications." *PLoS ONE* 4(7) (July 22):e6320. doi:10.1371/journal.pone.0006320.
17. Smith, Zachary J., Kaiqin Chu, Alyssa R. Espenson, Mehdi Rahimzadeh, Amy Gryshuk, Marco Molinaro, Denis M. Dwyre, Stephen Lane, Dennis Matthews, and Sebastian Wachsmann-Hogiu. 2011. "Cell-Phone-Based Platform for Biomedical Device Development and Education Applications." *PLoS ONE* 6(3) (March 2):e17150. doi:10.1371/journal.pone.0017150.
18. Wei, Qingshan, Hangfei Qi, Wei Luo, Derek Tseng, So Jung Ki, Zhe Wan, Zoltán Göröcs, et al. 2013. "Fluorescent Imaging of Single Nanoparticles and Viruses on a Smart Phone." *ACS Nano* (September 9). doi:10.1021/nn4037706. http://dx.doi.org/10.1021/nn4037706.
19. Banoo, Shabir, David Bell, Patrick Bossuyt, Alan Herring, David Mabey, Freddie Poole, Peter G. Smith, et al. 2006. "Evaluation of Diagnostic Tests for Infectious Diseases: General Principles." *Nature Reviews. Microbiology* 4(9 Suppl) (September):S21–S31. doi:10.1038/nrmicro1523.

20. Vasoo, Shawn, Jane Stevens, and Kamaljit Singh. 2009. "Rapid Antigen Tests for Diagnosis of Pandemic (Swine) Influenza A/H1N1." *Clinical Infectious Diseases: An Official Publication of the Infectious Diseases Society of America* 49(7) (October 1):1090–1093. doi:10.1086/644743.
21. Mills, Lisa A., Joseph Kagaayi, Gertrude Nakigozi, Ronald M. Galiwango, Joseph Ouma, Joseph P. Shott, Victor Ssempijja, et al. 2010. "Utility of a Point-of-Care Malaria Rapid Diagnostic Test for Excluding Malaria as the Cause of Fever Among HIV-Positive Adults in Rural Rakai, Uganda." *The American Journal of Tropical Medicine and Hygiene* 82(1) (January):145–147. doi:10.4269/ajtmh.2010.09-0408.
22. Wongsrichanalai, Chansuda, Mazie J. Barcus, Sinuon Muth, Awalludin Sutamihardja, and Walther H. Wernsdorfer. 2007. "A Review of Malaria Diagnostic Tools: Microscopy and Rapid Diagnostic Test (RDT)." *The American Journal of Tropical Medicine and Hygiene* 77(6 Suppl) (December):119–127.
23. Pattanasin, S., S. Proux, D. Chompasuk, K. Luwiradaj, P. Jacquier, S. Looareesuwan, and F. Nosten. 2003. "Evaluation of a New Plasmodium Lactate Dehydrogenase Assay (OptiMAL-IT®) for the Detection of Malaria." *Transactions of the Royal Society of Tropical Medicine and Hygiene* 97(6) (November 1):672–674. doi:10.1016/S0035-9203(03)80100-1.
24. Moody, A.H., and P.L. Chiodini. 2002. "Non-microscopic Method for Malaria Diagnosis Using OptiMAL IT, a Second-Generation Dipstick for Malaria pLDH Antigen Detection." *British Journal of Biomedical Science* 59(4): 228–231.
25. Moody, Anthony. 2002. "Rapid Diagnostic Tests for Malaria Parasites." *Clinical Microbiology Reviews* 15(1) (January) 66–78.
26. Alam, Mohammad Shafiul, Abu Naser Mohon, Shariar Mustafa, Wasif Ali Khan, Nazrul Islam, Mohammad Jahirul Karim, Hamida Khanum, David J. Sullivan Jr., and Rashidul Haque. 2011. "Real-Time PCR Assay and Rapid Diagnostic Tests for the Diagnosis of Clinically Suspected Malaria Patients in Bangladesh." *Malaria Journal* 10:175. doi:10.1186/1475-2875-10-175.
27. Gallegos, Dustin, Kenneth D. Long, Hojeong Yu, Peter P. Clark, Yixiao Lin, Sherine George, Pabitra Nath, and Brian T. Cunningham. 2013. "Label-free Biodetection Using a Smartphone." *Lab on a Chip* 13(11) (May 7): 2124–2132. doi:10.1039/C3LC40991K.
28. Lillehoj, Peter B., Ming-Chun Huang, Newton Truong, and Chih-Ming Ho. 2013. "Rapid Electrochemical Detection on a Mobile Phone." *Lab on a Chip* 13(15) (July 2):2950–2955. doi:10.1039/C3LC50306B.
29. Shen, Li, Joshua A. Hagen, and Ian Papautsky. 2012. "Point-of-care Colorimetric Detection with a Smartphone." *Lab on a Chip* 12(21) (November 7):4240–4243. doi:10.1039/c2lc40741h.
30. Oncescu, Vlad, Dakota O'Dell, and David Erickson. 2013. "Smartphone Based Health Accessory for Colorimetric Detection of Biomarkers in Sweat and Saliva." *Lab on a Chip* (June 19). doi:10.1039/C3LC50431J. http://pubs.rsc.org/en/content/articlelanding/2013/lc/c3lc50431j.
31. Preechaburana, Pakorn, Marcos Collado Gonzalez, Anke Suska, and Daniel Filippini. 2012. "Surface Plasmon Resonance Chemical Sensing on Cell Phones." *Angewandte Chemie International Edition* 51(46): 11585–11588. doi:10.1002/anie.201206804.
32. Ruano-López, Jesus M., Maria Agirregabiria, Garbiñe Olabarria, Dolores Verdoy, Dang D. Bang, Minqiang Bu, Anders Wolff, et al. 2009. "The SmartBioPhone, a Point of Care Vision under Development through Two European Projects: OPTOLABCARD and LABONFOIL." *Lab on a Chip* 9(11) (June 7):1495–1499. doi:10.1039/b902354m.

3 The Phone Oximeter

Christian Leth Petersen

CONTENTS

3.1 INTRODUCTION

The adoption of mobile phones in low- and middle-income countries is one of the most remarkable technology success stories in recent years. Areas that were not long ago without basic means of communication are now seeing substantial boosts to the local economies. The livelihoods of millions of people have improved as a result of the increased community connectivity, even as conventional infrastructure in many areas remains undeveloped.

A mobile phone is a sophisticated electronic device. It contains a powerful central processing unit, a flexible graphical user interface, and a high-quality analog–digital interface for performing voice calls and playing media files. While the majority of phones in low-income countries remain entry level "dumb" models, an increasing portion are smartphones capable of loading custom programs that can be downloaded from the Internet.

This new worldwide prevalence of handheld computing devices offers an unparalleled opportunity for improving health care in impoverished regions [1]. Past efforts to equip these areas with modern conventional hospital equipment have had little effect due to the lack of training, personnel, and elementary infrastructure, such as stable electrical power, to facilitate its use. Health care solutions delivered with use of mobile devices can circumvent many of these problems, and potentially reach people living in the most rural parts of the world.

Many of today's mobile phones are fitted with sensors for measuring acceleration, geo-location, lighting levels etc. The data from these sensors is available to programs running on the devices. If medical sensors measuring clinical data such as body temperature or blood oxygen saturation were integrated into the devices in the same way, we would have a new class of truly versatile personal diagnostic devices, that could radically change the way that health care is delivered.

Many efforts are currently underway to connect external medical devices to mobile phones, such as blood pressure monitors and blood glucose meters. Most of these devices are self-contained battery powered digital processing modules that communicate with the phone through Bluetooth radio signals or frequency keyed audio signals. The external hardware in such solutions is often redundant, as the phone itself is capable of powering and interfacing with the clinical sensors directly.

With a direct sensor interface, the phone acts not just as a display, but also as the sensor signal processing unit, making the sensor itself the only hardware external to the phone. This configuration reduces the cost of the solution to a minimum. This chapter discusses the implementation of such a direct interface to a pulse oximeter sensor for measuring the oxygen concentration in the blood, and considers many aspects of the system from interface design to signal processing and regulatory approval, accounting for recent and current work by the multi-disciplinary Pediatric Anesthesia Research Team of the University of British Columbia at BC Children's Hospital in Vancouver, Canada.

3.2 FUNDAMENTALS OF OXYGEN TRANSPORT IN THE BODY

Every cell in the human body needs oxygen. The harvesting of oxygen from the air and transport of oxygen through the body is a marvel of nature's engineering (Figure 3.1). Oxygen first enters the body through air inspired in the lungs. From here it enters capillaries in the thin walled alveoli sacs of the lungs by means of a gradient in the partial pressure of oxygen between the alveoli and the veins feeding the lung capillaries. Once inside the capillaries oxygen is captured by the red blood cells, which contains hemoglobin (Hb) molecules capable of binding to oxygen in a reversible process. The oxygenated hemoglobin molecule is called *oxy-hemoglobin* (HbO_2). The heart pumps the oxy-hemoglobin rich blood through the arteries to every part of the body, where the oxygen is metabolized by the cells.

This process of oxygen transport is critical to life. Without oxygen, even for short periods of time, our cells die, and extended loss of oxygen is fatal. The hemoglobin in the blood is normally almost fully saturated with oxygen. A decrease in oxygen content indicates that either the amount of oxygen being delivered throughout the body is reduced or the amount being consumed by the body is increased. For example, loss of oxygen supply will quickly lead to a drop in the concentration of oxy-hemoglobin in the blood. A number of respiratory [2] and cardiac diseases [3], as well as systemic diseases that affect multiple body systems including the lungs [4,5] also lower the oxygen content by interfering with different mechanisms in the oxygen transport pro-

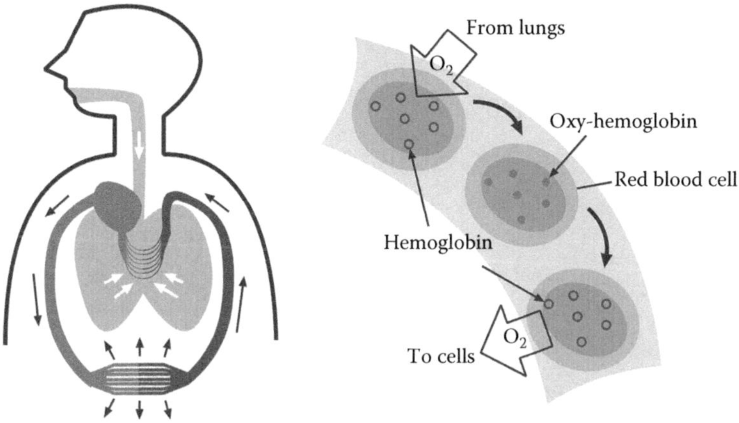

FIGURE 3.1 Oxygen transport fundamentals. Oxygen enters capillaries by gas exchange in the lungs, is reversibly bound to hemoglobin in the arterial blood and transported to the tissue, where it is metabolized. The de-oxygenized blood returns to the lungs through the veins, and the process repeats.

cess. Athletes experience drops in oxygen concentration during extreme exertions as their bodies momentarily use more oxygen than they can take in [6].

Hemoglobin and oxy-hemoglobin have markedly different optical spectra in the red and infrared range [7]. Hemoglobin-carrying oxygen (red blood) absorbs more infrared light and allows more red light to pass than hemoglobin without oxygen (blue blood) which allows more infrared light to pass. This is visible clinically by the skin turning blue after periods of oxygen desaturation. The optical effect offers a straightforward way to measure the concentration of oxygen in the blood noninvasively with a technology called *Pulse Oximetry.*

3.3 PULSE OXIMETRY

Pulse oximetry is a noninvasive diagnostic method that measures the proportion of hemoglobin in the blood that is actually carrying oxygen. This measure is known as *oxygen saturation* or SpO_2, and is expressed as a percentage of hemoglobin that has oxygen attached to it. One hundred percent oxygen saturation is attained when all the hemoglobin in the blood is completely saturated with oxygen.

A conventional pulse oximeter sensor shines two beams of red and infrared light through blood circulating in the small blood vessels of an extremity (e.g., a finger or ear), and detects the amount of transmitted light (Figure 3.2). The light beams are attenuated as they pass through the body, and the light intensity decreases exponentially with the path traveled, in accordance to the Beer–Lambert law:

$$I = I_0 10^{-\alpha l}, \tag{3.1}$$

where I is the transmitted intensity, I_0 is the incident intensity, l is the path length, and α is the absorption coefficient of blood and tissue at the particular wavelength of

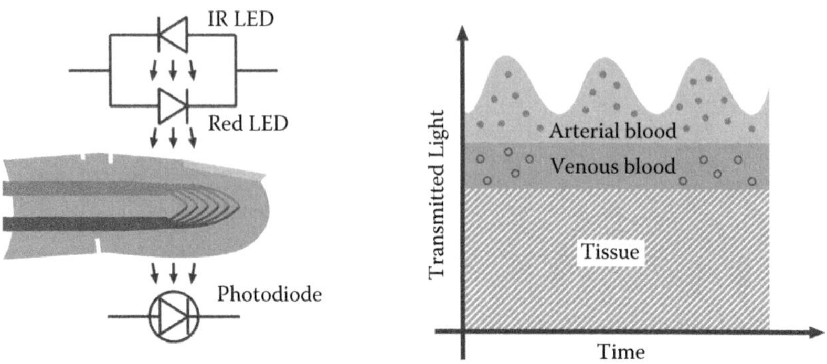

FIGURE 3.2 Principle of pulse oximetry. Red and infrared light-emitting diodes (LEDs) shine light through a body extremity such as a finger, and the transmitted light is detected by a photodiode. The arterial modulation of the transmitted light contains information about the relative amount of oxy-hemoglobin in the blood.

the incident light. By comparing the amount of light absorbed at two different wavelengths it is possible to calculate the oxygen saturation from the known difference in absorption spectra of hemoglobin and oxy-hemoglobin.

In the simplest interpretation, the signal from the sensor consists of a pulsatile component from the oxygen carrying arterial blood and a static component from venous blood and tissue (Figure 3.2). After separating the pulsatile (AC) and static (DC) components of the red and infrared oximeter signals, the normalized ratio of the red absorbance to the infrared absorbance can be expressed as:

$$R = \frac{\log_{10}(I_{AC+DC} / I_{DC})|_{\lambda_1}}{\log_{10}(I_{AC+DC} / I_{DC})|_{\lambda_2}}, \tag{3.2}$$

where λ_1 and λ_2 are the wavelengths of the red (660nm typ.) and infrared (890nm typ.) light, respectively.

In a real sensor, the light-emitting diodes (LEDs) emit not a single wavelength but a narrow band of wavelengths, typically with a half power spectral width of 30–50 nm, and the detector is a photodiode with a wavelength dependent sensitivity that is highest in the infrared region (Figure 3.3). Taking this into account, the measured signal from a diode with wavelength λ_1 can be estimated as:

$$I_{\lambda_1}(S) = \int_0^\infty i_{\lambda_1}(\lambda)s(\lambda)10^{(-\alpha_{HgO_2}(\lambda)S - \alpha_{Hg}(\lambda)(100-S))/100} d\lambda, \tag{3.3}$$

where $i_{\lambda_1}(\lambda)$ is the spectral intensity of the emitted light, $s(\lambda)$ is the spectral sensitivity of the detector, $\alpha_{Hg(O_2)}(\lambda)$ is the absorption coefficient of (oxy-)hemoglobin, and S is the oxygen saturation. We can use this expression to determine the relationship between R and S, through Equation (3.2), by numerical integration of the spectra in Figure 3.3.

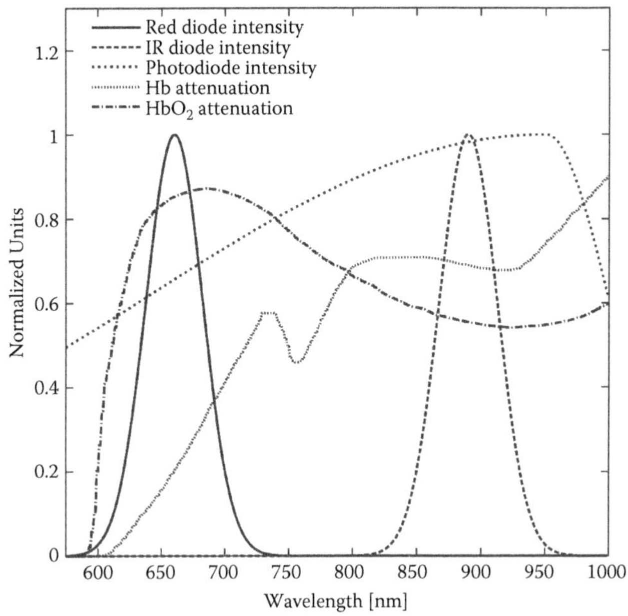

FIGURE 3.3 Spectral diode intensities, sensor sensitivity, and (oxy-)hemoglobin molar extinction coefficients for estimating the relative oxygen content in arterial blood.

The result of this calculation is shown as a solid line in Figure 3.4, along with an empirical comparison to a co-oximeter reference (i.e., invasive blood sampling). The general observed behavior is similar. However, the model does not give a very good fit to the real data. This is attributed to the presence of scattering phenomena in the tissue and sensor enclosure which are not accounted for in this simple model. A commonly quoted linear approximation to the ratio curve is [8]:

$$S = 110 - 25R, \tag{3.4}$$

also shown in Figure 3.4. The linear approximation does not give sufficiently accurate estimates of the oxygen saturation either. For this reason, clinical oximeters typically rely on lookup tables with the empirically determined calibration factors stored in the firmware of the instruments to produce accurate results. The calibration factors vary with sensor geometry, and most clinical sensors therefore incorporate an electronic identification that allows the oximeter instrument to select the lookup table appropriate for the particular sensor.

3.4 PULSE OXIMETRY AS A DIAGNOSTIC TOOL

Pulse oximetry may be used to detect reduced levels of oxygen in the blood before the clinical sign of oxygen deprivation (skin turns blue) can be seen. This early detection of a reduced level of oxygen allows early rescue before the oxygen concentration drops to critical levels. For this reason, pulse oximetry has contributed significantly

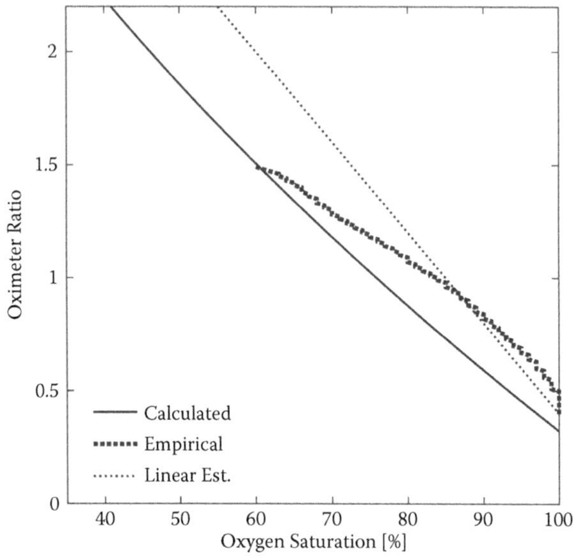

FIGURE 3.4 Relation between oximeter ratio and oxygen saturation based on calculations, measurements, and linear approximation.

to reducing the risk of death associated with anesthesia and surgery, and has become a standard monitoring device in modern hospitals [9,10]. Despite the importance to safety in anesthesia, many operating rooms in low- and middle-income countries are still not equipped with the devices. The World Health Organization (WHO) estimates a shortage of 90,000–150,000 oximeters in hospitals worldwide for anesthesia [11].

The pulse oximeter also has the potential to act as a diagnostic device for diseases that affect oxygen transport in the body, for example by impeding gas exchange in the failing lungs. Pulse oximetry can identify early signs of such diseases, monitor disease progression over time, and indicate disease severity. For example, decreased SpO_2 is a strong predictor of critical illness in respiratory diseases such as pneumonia and asthma [12–15], and other systemic infectious and inflammatory diseases [4]. Pneumonia diagnosis based on a low SpO_2 can differentiate severe pneumonia from mild respiratory tract infections such as the common cold.

Sepsis is an example of a serious inflammatory state of the body that affects the ability of the blood to carry oxygen, and is the final pathway for many common diseases such as pneumonia, malaria, and diarrhea. An estimated 7,500,000 children under the age of five die every year from these diseases, the majority as a consequence of sepsis [16]. Most of the deaths are due to a lack of timely diagnosis and treatment, and pulse oximetry could be a powerful clinical tool for early diagnosis and management, particularly in low- and middle-income countries where most deaths occur.

Unfortunately, conventional clinical pulse oximeters are expensive and bulky devices that are not of practical use in the areas where they would be clinically useful [17–19]. Leveraging the ubiquitous mobile phones as a diagnostic pulse oximetry platform could address this issue, and make this potentially life-saving technology widely available.

3.5 THE PHONE OXIMETER

To address the limited reach of conventional pulse oximetry, and make use of the prevalence of mobile phones, a clinical pulse oximeter sensor can be interfaced to a mobile phone (Figure 3.5). Commercially available pulse oximeter modules from Nonin and Masimo feature a UART communication interface and low power supply requirements which are directly compatible with smartphones. It is particularly easy

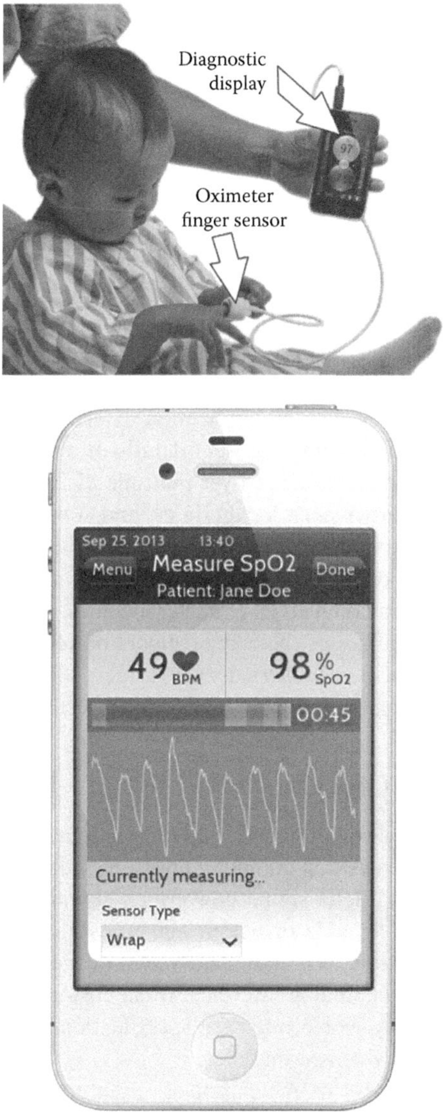

FIGURE 3.5 Elements of the phone oximeter. The phone oximeter consists of a clinical finger sensor interfaced to a smartphone running a custom application program. The screen shot shows a phone oximeter measurement in progress.

to interface these modules to the iPhone family of devices, as all the connections needed are readily accessible on the docking connector of the devices.

Starting from cardboard mockups of a mobile phone oximeter interface, created through discussions with the stakeholders and feedback from clinicians and anesthesia assistants, a user interface for a continuous mode pulse oximeter has been developed for use as a mobile anesthesia monitor [22]. This phone oximeter prototype application was written in a cross-platform development framework and deployed on iPod touch devices. The prototype was evaluated in usability studies combining think aloud task list completion with a standardized Mobile Phone Usability Questionnaire (MPUQ) [20,21]. The resulting overall acceptance rate was 81.9%, indicative that a phone-based oximeter is viable and indeed well received.

The prototype evolved into a set of full-featured oximeter research tools capable of recording high-quality pulse oximetry data [23] and capable of automatically transmitting the data to a remote clinical REDcap database [24] over a secure HTTPS connection on available Wifi networks. This suite of phone oximeter applications has been used successfully in eight separate clinical studies. To date, clinical data from more than 10,000 subjects in Canada, India, Bangladesh, Uganda, and South Africa has been collected with the applications.

Further work is currently being done to integrate the phone oximeter with the Pre-Eclampsia Integrated Estimate of RiSk (PIERS) model to estimate risk for adverse maternal outcomes [25]. The PIERS application extends the basic oximeter functionality with a data entry system to collect details of symptoms, medical history, and medications from a patient, taken over multiple visits [26]. The application is designed to be used by midwives in local clinics, and community health care workers in their regular visits to pregnant women's homes.

A limiting factor in the deployment of this first generation of phone oximeter implementations is the reliance on commercial oximeter modules. These are expensive redundant devices. The phone possesses the computational power to perform the necessary pulse oximetry signal processing internally. To achieve the lowest cost and highest degree of penetration, the oximeter sensor needs to be directly interfaced to the phone.

3.6 THE AUDIO PHONE OXIMETER

Mobile phones contain high-quality analog audio interfaces, which are a culmination of decades of evolution of desktop computer audio. Standard features of these interfaces include 24-bit sigma-delta signal converters, signal-to-noise ratios in excess of 90 dB, bandwidths of 48 kHz or better, and the ability of driving low impedance loads without distortion. The audio subsystem of the phone can be considered a generic high-performance analog interface. Most custom micro-controller sensor modules have considerably worse interface specifications, including those used in commercial pulse oximetry sensor modules.

Considering that the pulse oximeter sensor LEDs form a low impedance load (albeit non-linear) comparable to that of headphone speakers, and that the oximeter photodiode generates a signal comparable in magnitude to that of an electret microphone, it is possible that the audio interface of a smartphone can be put to service as a direct oximeter sensor interface. In doing so the redundant cost of an external micro-controller is eliminated, and the total cost of the new device is reduced to that of the finger probe itself.

The audio oximeter finger sensor is connected to the phone via the headset jack, a universal 3.5 mm four-conductor Tip-Ring-Ring-Sleeve (TRRS) connector present on all modern phones. The LEDs are connected between the tip and outer ring, and the photodiode between the sleeve and inner ring of the connector (Figure 3.6) [27–29].

The LEDs of the oximeter sensor are driven by the speaker output of the phone. The diodes of conventional oximeter sensors are wired in reverse polarity, which facilitates activating the diodes at opposite polarities of the driving audio signal. The forward voltages of the LEDs are approximately 1.3 V and 1.8 V for the infrared and red emitter, respectively. In the case of an iPhone smartphone or equivalent, the maximum

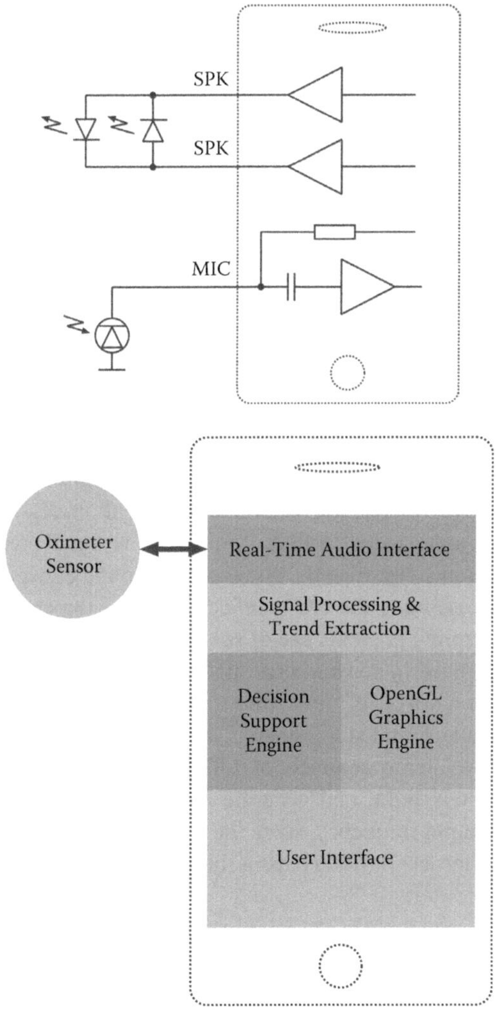

FIGURE 3.6 Schematic of the audio phone oximeter electrical interface (top), and block diagram of the software interface components (bottom).

peak-to-peak amplitude of the stereo audio output signal is in excess of 2 V, and sufficient to drive the diodes without any conditioning or voltage boosting circuitry.

The sensor photodiode generates a voltage in response to the transmitted light in the sensor. This signal is compatible with the microphone input of the audio channel, and can be detected without amplification or conditioning. It was however found beneficial to boost the signal amplitude with a single field-effect transistor powered by the microphone bias signal, to improve performance under low transmissibility conditions.

As the oximeter finger sensor is interfaced directly to the phone, all signal processing must be implemented in software and be designed to operate with AC only signals, which is a requirement for an audio-based system. This can be accomplished with the same real-time audio Application Programming Interface (API) that is used for Voice-Over-IP (VOIP) and similar applications requiring full-duplex low latency sound processing. This API provides low-level access points to the synchronized input and output channels needed by the oximeter signal processing algorithms.

Once the raw input signal has been converted into numeric trends for oxygen saturation and heart rate, the trend values can in turn be fed to a decision support engine for higher order alerts and diagnostic output. The flexibility and power of the processing unit on mobile phones and the high data sampling rate provides new opportunities for novel signal processing paradigms and diagnostic capabilities that can enhance the usability and signal quality.

3.7 NOVEL OXYGEN SATURATION ALGORITHMS

Conventional oximeter signal processing is performed by embedded micro controllers or digital signal processors that often have limited performance and computational capabilities. The audio phone oximeter can draw on the much more powerful general purpose processor onboard the phone for signal processing. This can be leveraged to implement more accurate algorithms and new signal processing paradigms.

The biggest difference between the audio oximeter and conventional oximeters in terms of signal processing is the AC coupled nature of the electrical interface. For example, the AC coupling prevents use of square waveforms and sampling on signal plateaus, commonly used in conventional algorithms.

As an example of a novel AC algorithm for extracting oxygen saturation, we can consider sending a sinusoidal stereophonic signal to the LEDs with a phase difference between the two stereo channels of 180 degrees (Figure 3.7). This will cause the LEDs to alternately light, and generate a monophonic input signal containing peaks at twice the output frequency, since the red and infrared LEDs of the oximeter sensor activate on alternate half-periods of the output waveform. We can express the sinusoidal output as:

$$O_1 = A\sin(\omega t),\ O_2 = -A\sin(\omega t), \tag{3.5}$$

where A is the amplitude of the outgoing waveform, ω is the angular frequency, and t is time. The incoming waveform signal can be approximated by positive sine half cycles of differing amplitude:

$$I = \left\{ \frac{1}{2} I_{Red} \left(\mathrm{sq}(\omega t) + 1 \right) + \frac{1}{2} I_{IR} \left(1 - \mathrm{sq}(\omega t) \right) \right\} \sin(\omega t), \tag{3.6}$$

where I_{Red} and I_{IR} are the amplitudes of the signals from each diode, and sq(ωt) is a square waveform of Fourier expansion:

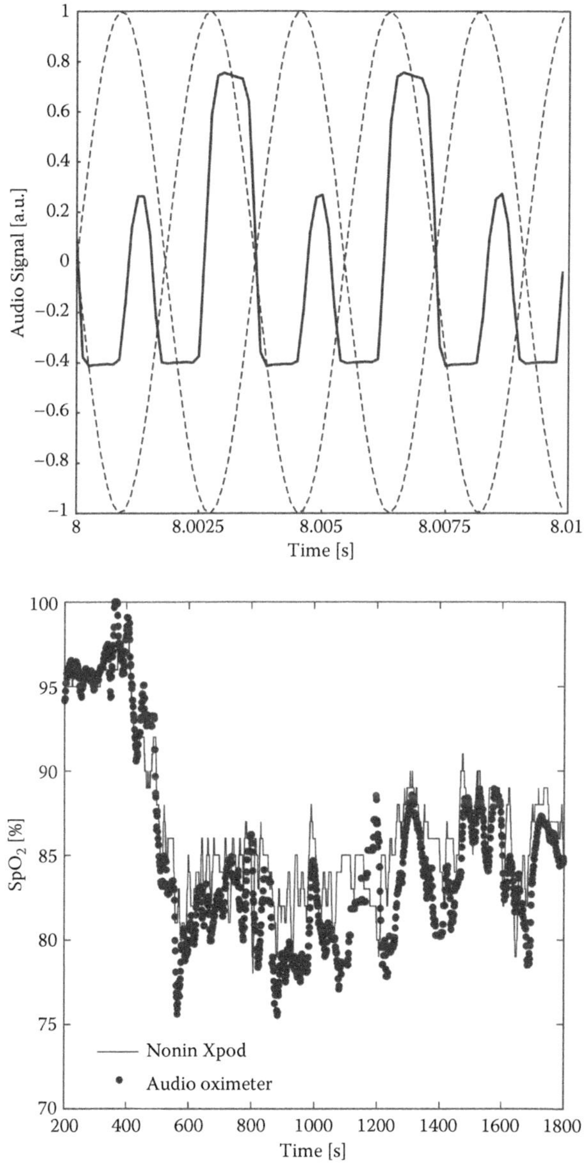

FIGURE 3.7 Top: example of audio oximeter driving signals (dashed) and frequency-doubled input signal (solid). Bottom: comparison of oxygen saturation output of the quadrature decoder algorithm (bullets) with readings from a commercial oximeter (solid).

$$\mathrm{sq}(u) = \frac{4}{\pi}\sum_{k=1}^{\infty}\frac{\sin((2k-1)u)}{2k-1}. \tag{3.7}$$

Expression (3.6) can be simplified to:

$$I = \frac{1}{2}(I_{Red} + I_{IR})\sin(\omega t) + \frac{1}{2}(I_{Red} - I_{IR})\mathrm{sq}(\omega t)\sin(\omega t). \tag{3.8}$$

Quadrature demodulation can be performed on this input waveform, at angular frequencies ω and 2ω, followed by low pass filtering. This will eliminate all higher harmonics of the square waveform. The amplitude of the demodulated quantities are:

$$I_{\omega} = \frac{1}{4}(I_{Red} + I_{IR}), \tag{3.9}$$

and

$$I_{2\omega} = \frac{1}{2\pi}(I_{Red} - I_{IR}). \tag{3.10}$$

I_{Red} and I_{IR} can now be determined from these demodulated quantities:

$$I_{Red} = 2I_w + \pi I_{2w}, \tag{3.11}$$

and

$$I_{IR} = 2I_w - \pi I_{2w}. \tag{3.12}$$

The static (DC) and dynamic (AC) component of each waveform can be extracted by conventional oximeter signal processing methods, and the oxygen saturation ratio derived from

$$R = \frac{I_{Red}^{AC} / I_{Red}^{DC}}{I_{IR}^{AC} / I_{IR}^{DC}}. \tag{3.13}$$

The oxygen saturation is finally determined by lookup in a calibration table as described in Section 3.3. To compare the new algorithm with a conventional commercial oximeter we collected data simultaneously from the audio oximeter and a Nonin Xpod oximeter on an Apple iPod touch device while a subject entered a normobaric (sea level atmosphere) hypoxia (low oxygen) chamber, leading to a sudden drop in oxygen saturation (Figure 3.7). Good agreement was found between the output of the two devices.

Conventional algorithms for extraction of oxygen saturation can also be used with the audio oximeter, and the high sampling rate of the audio channel can impact these algorithms favorably. For example, in reference [33], the raw red and infrared signals were band-pass filtered by a fourth-order Butterworth filter with lower and upper cutoff frequencies of 0.5 Hz and 5 Hz, and the filtered signal used for peak detection, using a simple level-based algorithm. The detected peaks triggered the calculation of oxygen saturation using standard techniques.

3.8 NOVEL HEART RATE ALGORITHMS

Most conventional heart rate detection algorithms can be used in the audio oximeter, though many require computationally intensive filtering to provide accurate results. In many cases, fast algorithms can take advantage of the high sampling rate of the audio channel to provide sufficiently accurate results [30,31].

For example, as a novel algorithm that allows high-speed detection of heart rate, we can consider a simple one-dimensional iterative function of form:

$$f_n = \begin{cases} \frac{1}{2}(1 - f_{n-1}), & \text{if } P_n > P_{n-1} \\ \frac{1}{2} f_{n-1}, & \text{if } P_n \leq P_{n-1} \end{cases},$$

where P_n represents the photoplethysmogram waveform samples. This is a non-linear scaling invariant function that effectively converts the waveform to a rapidly switching normalized signal. The function converges exponentially to 1 when approaching a peak, and drops below 0.5 instantly after the peak. This can be used for a very simple and fast peak detection algorithm (Figure 3.8).

This algorithm was implemented in the C programming language and applied to unfiltered annotated plethysmogram benchmark data from pediatric subjects with 15,868 visually marked peaks [31]. No tuning or peak position validation was done against the benchmark data set. Peak detection thresholds were determined on independent data. Statistical analysis revealed positive predictive value of 98.6–99.8% and sensitivity of 97.3–98.1%, which is adequate for most applications.

Good agreement was found when comparing the output of this algorithm with that of the Nonin Xpod commercial oximeter (Figure 3.8). The dynamic response is slightly different as the time constants of two signal processing algorithms differ.

Conventional time- or frequency-domain heart rate algorithms can also be used on the audio oximeter data. The versatile mobile platforms offer great freedom to choose the algorithms that suit the application best. In cases where the signal processing quota must be limited, a simple algorithm like the above may provide a clinically acceptable tradeoff between speed and accuracy.

3.9 REGULATORY VALIDATION

Any device that provides information used for diagnostic purposes in humans falls under regulatory control. It is essential for the success of any new mobile medical sensing technology that regulatory requirements be considered and addressed. The regulations around mobile health care solutions are still in their infancy and likely to change significantly in the coming years.

Data: Raw plethysmogram value P_n
Result: Peak marker bloolean *peak*

F_n: *iterative function fractal*
begin
  if $P_n > P_{n-1}$ then
    $f_n = \frac{1}{2}(1 + f_{n-1})$
  else
    $f_n = \frac{1}{2} f_{n-1}$
  end
  if $f_n < 0.6$ and $f_{n-1} > 0.999$ then
    $peak = True$
  else
    $peak = False$
  end
  $P_{n-1} \longleftarrow P_n$
  $f_{n-1} \longleftarrow f_n$
end

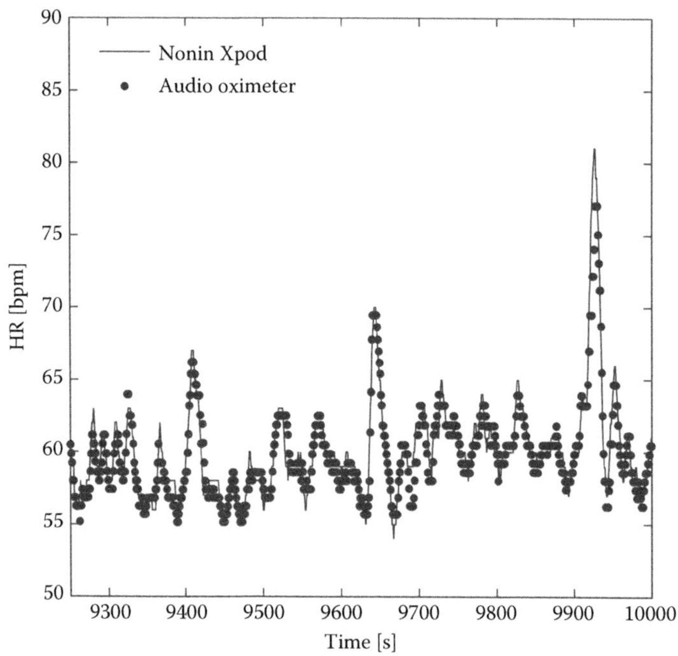

FIGURE 3.8 Top: fast heart rate detection algorithm. Bottom: comparing the fast heart rate algorithm (bullets) with readings from a commercial Nonin Xpod oximeter module (solid).

A clinical phone oximeter must adhere to both general medical device requirements and pulse oximeter specific standards. In particular, the ISO pulse oximeter standard requires the root-mean-square error, A_{RMS}, to be less than 4% with respect to co-oximeter blood gas readings [32]. The standard permits validation against a single approved oximeter as secondary standard. Independent of the ISO standards, the WHO has a stricter requirement of $A_{RMS} < 2\%$ [11].

In a first step toward verifying regulatory compliance of the audio oximeter, we have performed an adult volunteer observational study in a normobaric hypoxia chamber with ethics approval and informed consent [33]. In this study data was recorded using iPhone 3G and 3GS devices and two clinical pulse oximeter sensors attached to two fingers on the subjects' non-dominant hands (Figure 3.9). The first sensor was connected directly to the audio port of the iPhone, and the second to a commercially available (FDA approved) Nonin Xpod pulse oximeter module interfaced through the iPhone docking connector.

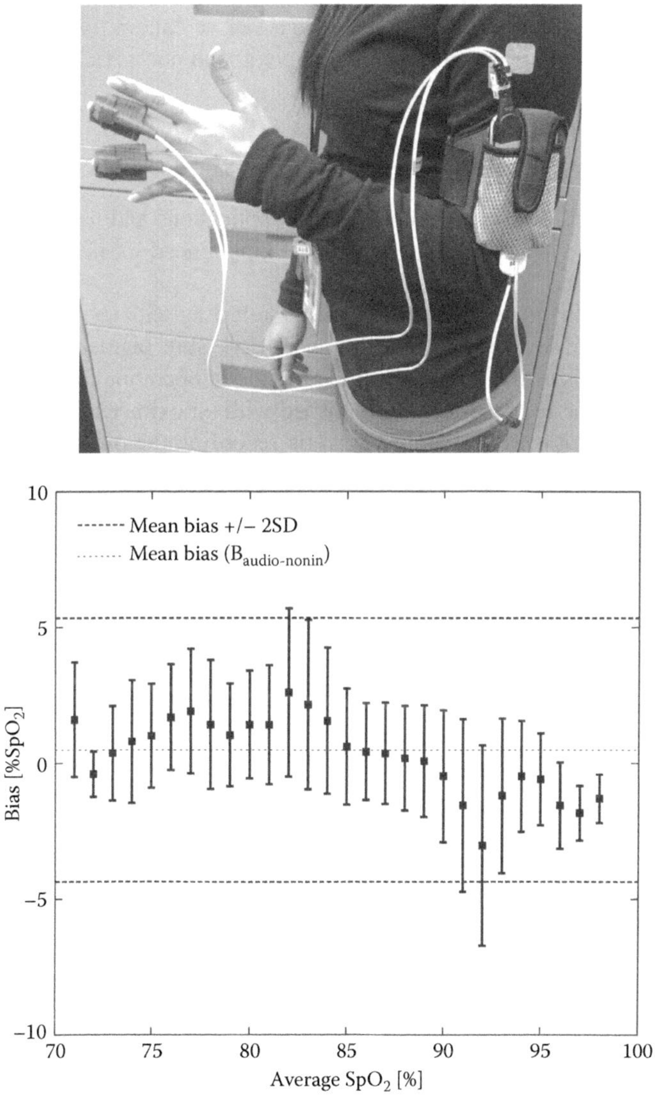

FIGURE 3.9 Audio oximeter and Nonin Xpod reference mobile device setup (top) and Bland–Altman plot showing the performance of the audio-based phone oximeter (bottom).

SpO_2 and pulse rate readings from the Nonin module and the raw red and infrared pulse oximetry data from the audio sensor were simultaneously recorded and used to estimate A_{RMS} using the Nonin module as a secondary standard. The audio oximeter was found to have an RMS accuracy with respect to the Nonin device of 2.47%. The Nonin device states 2% RMS accuracy against blood gas readings. The audio oximeter net accuracy with respect to blood gas readings is therefore $\sqrt{2.0^2 + 2.47^2} = 3.18\%$, within the accepted ISO range.

Overall, Bland–Altman representation of the data shows a good performance over the full range of clinically relevant saturation values (Figure 3.9). The apparent deviation at values of 91% and 92% is due to a lack of data in this region. The data collected in the study was predominantly hypoxic and normoxic, with limited data in the intermediate range.

3.10 SYSTEMATIC VERIFICATION

The emerging field of clinical mobile health applications and the reliance on consumer electronics for medical diagnosis is creating a need for new methods of systematic verification.

In the case of the phone oximeter, systematic testing with respect to low peripheral perfusion and low optical transmittance (dark skin pigmentation) is of most importance, as this is the most challenging regime of operation for pulse oximeters.

Such systematic tests can be accomplished with an oximeter simulator. By controlling the simulator with a computer while recording the output from the phone oximeter, the oximeter performance can be determined without expensive and time consuming human trials [34,35]. With a suitable visual representation that reflects the ISO standard requirements for pulse oximetry, performance can be confirmed immediately by inspection (Figure 3.10), and oxygen saturation levels can be tested that would otherwise be unsafe and unethical to reach in human trials.

Using this systematic verification approach, the audio oximeter was found to give good readings down to perfusion of about 1% at transmission levels down to 0.5%, sufficient to provide readings on subjects with low perfusion and dark skin pigmentation.

3.11 BEYOND CONVENTIONAL PULSE OXIMETRY

A pulse oximeter sensor is a versatile and safe device that provides information about pulsatile blood. The noninvasive nature of the sensor makes it an ideal platform for extracting information beyond oxygen saturation and heart rate.

For example, substances other than oxy-hemoglobin, such as carboxy-hemoglobin created when carbon monoxide binds to hemoglobin, also absorb light and can be detected by the same principles used in a conventional oximeter. This requires measurements at additional wavelengths in order to separate the signals from multiple substances. Multi-wavelength technology can also be used to extract the total hemoglobin content in the blood, an important clinical measure.

The pulse oximeter sensor can also potentially be used to assess capillary refill time (CRT). CRT is the rate at which blood refills empty capillaries, and is usually

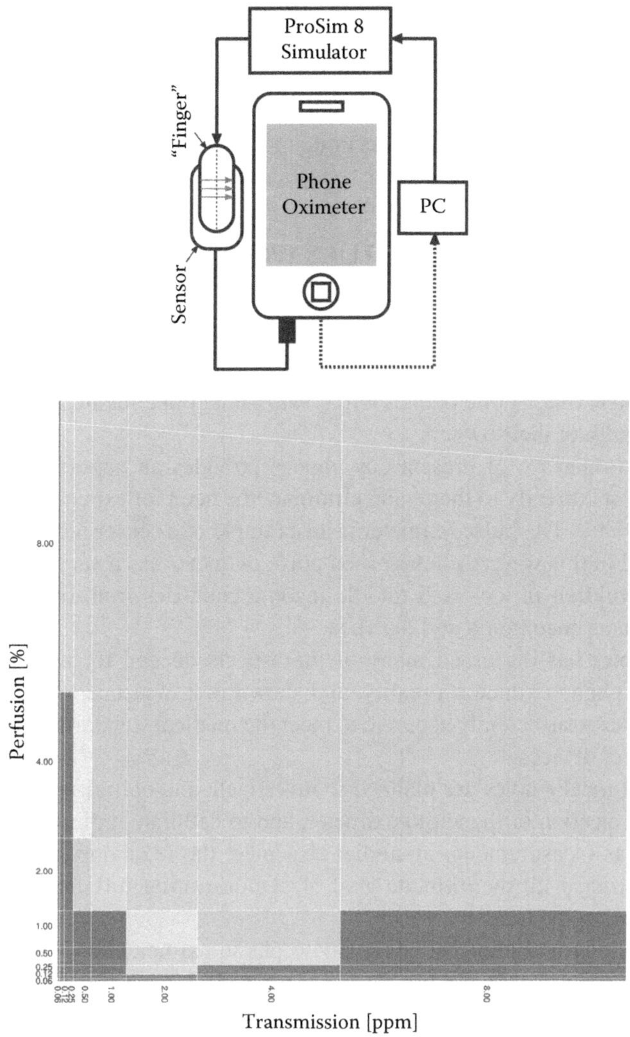

FIGURE 3.10 Automated simulation setup (top) and automatically generated map of low-perfusion and low transmission performance (bottom). The graded gray scale corresponds to the maximum of oxygen saturation bias and standard deviation; with 0% being light gray and > = 4% being dark gray (From Petersen C. et al. Systematic Evaluation of Mobile Phone Pulse Oximetry. American Society of Anesthesiologists (ASA) Annual Meeting abstracts, San Francisco, CA, 2013. With permission.)

measured by pressing on the nail bit of a finger or toe until it turns white, and noting the time it takes for the color to return. CRT is typically not measured with great precision. A phone oximeter application can potentially be used to make better quantitative measurements, by prompting users to press the oximeter finger probe for a specific interval and analyzing the oximeter waveform to determine the refill time in a much more reproducible way than previously possible [36,37]. This can potentially increase the usefulness of the CRT as a diagnostic tool in critical care.

The powerful user interface of the phone can also be used to collect information about the patient such as demographics and medical history that can be combined with the sensor readings to provide accurate medical diagnosis and treatment advice not possible with a conventional pulse oximeter alone.

3.12 CONCLUSION AND FUTURE WORK

The global availability of mobile phones has opened a new exciting chapter in the delivery of health care. The platforms hold promise of not only serving as a means of communication, but of performing clinical sensing at the community level. In the future it is likely that mobile phones will contain integrated medical sensors that can assess the health of their owners.

The audio interface of present day phones provides an opportunity to connect medical sensors directly to them, and eliminate the need for expensive external processing hardware. The pulse oximeter is an example of a sensor technology that can be interfaced in this way. A phone-based pulse oximeter has a very real potential of preventing children in low- and middle-income countries from dying of common diseases such as pneumonia and diarrhea.

This chapter has discussed many of the aspects needed for making a clinical audio-based phone oximeter a reality, and shown first evidence to support that the audio oximeter is sufficiently accurate to meet the medical standard requirements for pulse oximeter devices.

Further clinical studies are planned to investigate and optimize the performance and artifact rejection of the audio oximeter, and to calibrate it directly against invasive blood gas measurements in studies that meet the regulatory requirements for oximeter testing, with the ultimate goal of demonstrating full compliance to both ISO and WHO standards.

The simplicity and low cost of the audio phone oximeter and the close correlation to approved clinical solutions promises an exciting new path for disseminating diagnostic tools to the furthest regions of the world.

REFERENCES

1. The United Nations Foundation, and Vodafone Partnership. mHealth for Development: The Opportunity of Mobile Technology for Healthcare in the Developing World, 2009. http://www.unfoundation.org/what-we-do/issues/global-health/mhealth-report.html, accessed April 16, 2014.
2. Neuman M.I., Monuteaux M.C., Scully K.J., Bachur R.G. Prediction of pneumonia in a pediatric emergency department. *Pediatrics*, vol. 128, no. 2, August 2011, pp. 246–53.
3. Thangaratinam S., Brown K., Zamora J., Khan K.S., Ewer A.K. Pulse oximetry screening for critical congenital heart defects in asymptomatic newborn babies: A systematic review and meta-analysis. *The Lancet*, vol. 6736, no. 12, May 2012.
4. Duke T., Blaschke J., Sialis S., Bonkowsky J.L. Hypoxaemia in acute respiratory and non-respiratory illnesses in neonates and children in a developing country. *Archives of Disease in Childhood*, vol. 86, no. 2, February 2002, pp. 108–12.

5. Subhi R., Adamson M., Campbell H., Weber M., Smith K., Duke T. The prevalence of hypoxaemia among ill children in developing countries: A systematic review. *The Lancet Infectious Diseases*, vol. 9, no. 4, April 2009, pp. 219–27.
6. Billaut F., Smith K. Prolonged repeated-sprint ability is related to arterial O_2 desaturation in men. *Int J Sports Physiol Perform*, vol. 5, 2010, pp. 197–209.
7. Prahl, S.A. A compendium of tissue optical properties. http://omlc.ogi.edu/spectra/hemoglobin, accessed April 16, 2014.
8. Rusch T.L., Sankar R., Scharf J.E. Signal processing methods for pulse oximetry. *Computers in Biology and Medicine*, vol. 26, 1996, pp. 143–159
9. Eichhorn J.H., Cooper J.B., Cullen D.J., Maier W.R., Philip J.H., Seeman R.G. Standards for patient monitoring during anesthesia at Harvard Medical School. *JAMA*, vol. 256, 1986, p. 1017–20.
10. Gibbs N., Rodoreda P. Anaesthetic mortality rates in Western Australia 1980–2002. *Anaesthesia and Intensive Care*, vol. 33, 2005, p. 61622.
11. WHO Global Pulse Oximetry Project, First International Consultation Meeting, Geneva, CH, 2008.
12. Madico G. et al. The role of pulse oximetry. Its use as an indicator of severe respiratory disease in Peruvian children living at sea level. *Arch. Pediatr. Adolesc. Med.*, vol. 149, 1995, pp. 1259–1263.
13. Rosen L.M., Yamamoto L.G., Wiebe R. A. Pulse oximetry to identify a high-risk group of children with wheezing. *Am J Emerg Med*, vol. 7, no. 6, November 1989, pp. 567–570.
14. Fu L.Y. et al. Brief hospitalization and pulse oximetry for predicting amoxicillin treatment failure in children with severe pneumonia. *Pediatrics*, vol. 118, no. 6, December 2006, pp. e1822–e1830.
15. Majumdar S.R., Eurich D.T., Gamble J.M., Senthilselvan, A., Marrie T.J. Oxygen saturations less than 92% are associated with major adverse events in outpatients with pneumonia: A population-based cohort study. *Clinical Infectious Diseases: An official Publication of the Infectious Diseases Society of America*, vol. 52, no. 3, February 2011, pp. 325–331.
16. Wiens M.O., Kumbakumba E., Kissoon N., Ansermino J.M., Ndamira A., Larson C.P. Pediatric sepsis in the developing world: Challenges in defining sepsis and issues in post-discharge mortality. *Clin Epidemiol.* vol. 4, 2012, pp. 319–325.
17. Hansen D., Gausi S.C., Merikebu M. Anaesthesia in Malawi: Complications and deaths. *Tropical Doctor*, vol. 30, 2000, pp. 146–149.
18. Ouro-Bangna Maman A.F., Tomta K., Ahouangbvi S., Chobli M. Deaths associated with anaesthesia in Togo, West Africa. *Tropical Doctor*, vol 35, 2005, pp. 220–222.
19. Heywood A.J., Wilson I.H., Sinclair J.R. Perioperative mortality in Zambia. *Annals of the Royal College of Surgeons of England*, vol 71, 1989, pp. 354–358.
20. Ryu, Y.S. Mobile phone usability questionnaire (MPUQ) and automated usability evaluation. *Human-Computer Interaction*, Part I, HCII 2009, LNCS 5610, 2009, pp. 349–351.
21. Karlen W., Dumont G., Petersen C., Gow J., Lim J., Sleiman J., Ansermino J.M. Human-centered phone oximeter interface design for the operating room. Proceedings of the International Conference on Health Informatics, Rome, Italy, 2011, pp. 433–438.
22. Karlen W., Hudson J., Petersen C., Anand R., Dumont G.A., Ansermino J.M. The phone oximeter. Unconference of the IEEE Engineering in Medicine and Biology Society, August 30, Boston, 2011.
23. Dunsmuir D., Petersen C., Karlen W., Lim J., Dumont G.A., Ansermino J.M. The phone oximeter for mobile spot-check. Society for Technology in Anesthesia 2012 Annual Meeting, Palm Beach, FL, January 18–21, 2012.

24. Harris P.A., Taylor R., Thielke R., Payne J., Gonzalez N., Conde J.G. Research electronic data capture (REDCap)—A metadata-driven methodology and workflow process for providing translational research informatics support. *J Biomed Inform.* vol. 42(2), 2009, pp. 377–381.
25. von Dadelszen P., Payne B., Li J., Ansermino J.M., Broughton-Pipkin F., Cote A.M., Douglas J.M., Gruslin A., Hutcheon J.A., Joseph K.S., Kyle P.M., Lee T., Loughna P., Menzies J.M., Merialdi M., Millman A.L., Moore M.P., Moutquin J.M., Ouellet A.B., Smith G.N., Walker J.J., Walley K.R., Walters B.N., Widmer M., Lee S.K., Russell J.A., Magee L.A. Predicting adverse maternal outcomes in pre-eclampsia: The fullPIERS (Pre-eclampsia Integrated Estimate of RiSk) model—development and validation. *Lancet*, vol. 377(9761), 2011, pp. 219–227.
26. Dunsmuir D.T., Payne B.A., Cloete G., Petersen C.L., Görges M., Lim J., von Dadelszen P., Dumont G.A., Ansermino J.M. Development of mHealth Applications for preeclampsia triage. *IEEE Journal of Biomedical and Health Informatics,* Vol PP, Issue 99, Page 1.
27. Petersen C. Implementing the phone oximeter. Pulse Oximetry, Anesthesia and Beyond Workshop, Vancouver, BC, May 19–20, 2011.
28. Petersen C.L., Ansermino J.M., Dumont G.A. Audio phone oximeter. *Society of Technology in Anesthesia*, West Palm Beach, Florida, 2012.
29. Petersen C., Gan H., Ansermino J.M., Dumont G.A. Comparing a new ultra-low cost pulse oximeter with two commercial oximeters. IAMPOV International Symposium, Yale University, New Haven, June 29–July 1, 2012.
30. Karlen W., Petersen C., Gow J., Ansermino J.M., Dumont G.A. An adaptive single frequency phase vocoder for low-power heart rate detection. BIODEVICES 2011—Proceedings of the International Conference on Biomedical Electronics and Devices, Rome, Italy, January 26–29, 2011, pp. 30–35.
31. Petersen C., Ansermino J.M., Dumont G.A. High-speed algorithm for plethysmograph peak detection in real-time applications. Society for Technology in Anesthesia 2012 Annual Meeting, Palm Beach, FL, January 18–21, 2012.
32. ISO 80601-2-61 Medical electrical equipment Part 2-61: Particular requirements for basic safety and essential performance of pulse oximeter equipment. Geneva, Switzerland, 2011.
33. Petersen C., Gan H., MacInnis M.J., Dumont G.A., Ansermino J.M. Ultra-low-cost clinical pulse oximetry. Annual International Conference of the IEEE Engineering in Medicine and Biology Society, Osaka, Japan, 2013, pp. 2874–2877.
34. Petersen C., Gan H., Görges M., Dumont G.A. Ansermino J.M. Systematic evaluation of mobile phone pulse oximetry. American Society of Anesthesiologists (ASA) Annual Meeting abstracts, San Francisco, CA, 2013.
35. Petersen C., Chen T.P., Ansermino J.M., Dumont G.A. Design and evaluation of a low-cost smartphone pulse oximeter. *Sensors*, vol. 13, 2013, pp. 16882–16893.
36. Karlen W., Pickard A., Daniels J., Kwizera A., Ibingira C., Dumont G.A., Ansermino J.M. Automated validation of capillary refill time measurements using photo-plethysmogram from a portable device for effective triage in children. Proceedings of the 2010 IEEE Global Humanitarian Technology Conference, Seattle, 2010, pp. 66–71.
37. Karlen W., Petersen C., Pickard A., Dumont G., Ansermino J.M. Capillary refill time assessment using a mobile phone application (iRefill). American Society of Anesthesiologists (ASA) Annual Meeting abstracts, 2010.

4 Current Technology and Advances in Transepidermal Water Loss Sensors

Pietro Salvo, Bernardo Melai, Nicola Calisi, and Fabio Di Francesco

CONTENTS

4.1 INTRODUCTION: TRANSEPIDERMAL WATER LOSS (TEWL)

The skin is an organ with twofold functionality. It prevents the loss of internal fluids and provides a protective barrier against exogenous agents that may damage or alter the biological functions of an organism. Nevertheless, skin is permeable to water molecules through a passive diffusion process called *transepidermal water loss* (TEWL), which is not to be confused with sensible perspiration as it excludes the excretions of sweat glands. However, in the literature, the same terminology often refers to the total amount of water loss through the skin. TEWL mainly depends on the external environment relative humidity and temperature, and on the thickness and integrity of the *stratum corneum*, the uppermost layer of epidermis [1].

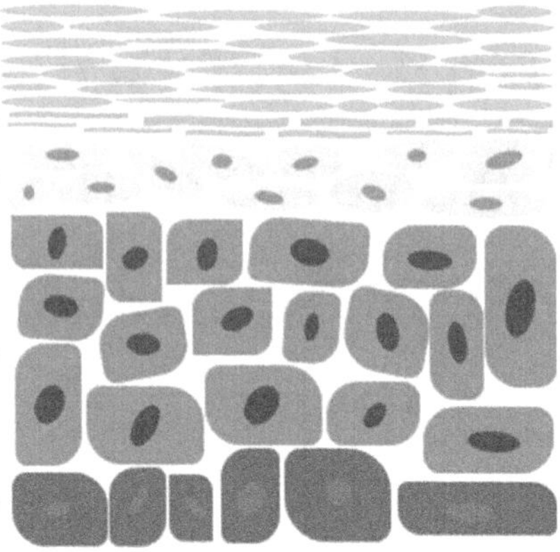

FIGURE 4.1 Structure of epidermis. *Stratum lucidum* is present only in palms and soles.

Epidermis is the outermost stratum of the skin and is composed of four layers, except in palms and soles where there is a fifth layer called the *stratum lucidum*. Figure 4.1 shows the epidermis and the main tasks of the stratum corneum [2].

TEWL is measured in g/(m^2·h) and, for healthy skin in adults, normal values range between 4 and 8 g/(m^2·h) [3]. In dermatology and cosmetology, TEWL is a relevant factor because it is an index of the health condition of the skin. A diminished function in the skin barrier corresponds to an increase in the TEWL value, which thus can vice versa be associated to skin damage. For example, in burns or granulating wounds, water loss may exceed 140 and 200 g/(m^2·h), respectively [4]. Augmented TEWL values are observed in case of *ichthyosis*, atopic dermatitis, and psoriasis, or can be associated to physical and chemical agents that disrupt the skin normal conditions [5,6]. TEWL is also influenced by other elements: endogenous factors such as age, gender, and circadian rhythm can lead to significant variations; minor fluctuations are also associated to air convection and light [5]. Therefore, a reliable measurement technique has to include and weigh the contributions of these possible interferences. This is particularly important because the TEWL measurement is always indirect since, being a property of the skin, it can only be evaluated by calculating the evaporation rate in a volume adjacent to a body part.

This chapter provides an overlook of the most common existing techniques and instruments to achieve a coherent understanding of the TEWL measurement. New technologies that can be implemented in the near future for developing portable and wearable TEWL sensors are also presented.

4.2 CURRENT TECHNOLOGIES FOR TRANSEPIDERMAL WATER LOSS SENSORS

4.2.1 Theory

In 1977, Nilsson published a seminal paper to measure the water exchange through skin [7]. His method is widely adopted in the commercially available TEWL instruments. Supposing that there is no thermal diffusion and forced convection, the water exchange through a stationary water-permeable surface can be derived from the vapor-pressure gradient contiguous to the surface. From Fick's first law of diffusion, in one-dimensional space, x, there is a proportionality between the vapor flow density J [mass· length^{-2}·time^{-1}] and the vapor pressure gradient ΔP along x:

$$J \propto \frac{\Delta P}{\Delta x} \tag{4.1}$$

The proportionality constant is known as the *diffusion coefficient*, D, expressed in [length^{2}·time^{-1}]. Therefore,

$$J = D \cdot \frac{\Delta P}{\Delta x} \tag{4.2}$$

D is usually set as constant, but it depends on temperature and atmospheric pressure. Although the maximum variations are in the order of ±6% and can be neglected for TEWL measurement, for very precise measurement the following expression for D can be used [8]:

$$D = D_0 \left(\frac{T}{T_0}\right)^n \frac{p_0}{p} \tag{4.3}$$

where T is the actual temperature in Kelvin, *n* is 1.5 for water vapor diffusion in air, $T_0 = 273.16$ K, $p_0 = 760$ mmHg, $D_0 = 0.219$ cm^2/s, and *p* is the vapor pressure. Nilsson's main achievement is to assume that the value of the gradient is approximately proportional to the difference between the vapor pressures measured at two separate fixed points located on a line perpendicular to the surface of the skin. It follows that the problem of measuring TEWL reduces to the calculus of the vapor pressure or, in other words, of the relative humidity (RH) values at two points close to the skin. In fact, at each point, the vapor pressure can be calculated as $RH \cdot p_{SAT}$, where p_{SAT} is the water vapor saturation pressure that can be straightforwardly obtained, if the temperature is known, by Antoine equation [9]. As described in [10], the ratio $\Delta x/D$ can be defined as a diffusion resistance R. The inverse of R is called *permeability*. Substituting R in Equation (4.1), it follows:

$$J = \frac{\Delta P}{\mathrm{R}} \tag{4.4}$$

which is a different formulation of the Ohm's law for the water exchange through the skin.

Guidelines for a proper measurement of TEWL are described in [11] and [12]. It is recommended to perform the measurement in a controlled environment at temperature and RH in the range 20–22°C and 40–60%, respectively. The subject under test should acclimatize for 15 to 30 min before starting the measurement to reduce inaccuracies due to abrupt changes in environmental conditions. Preferably, the probe should be placed on the volar forearm, i.e., on the same side as the palm of the hand, not close to the wrist.

4.2.2 Open Chamber

Nilsson's method is known as the *open chamber* method because the measurement chamber is essentially a hollow cylinder where one side is in contact with the skin, while the other is open to let the water vapor diffuse in the external environment (Figure 4.2).

One of the first pioneering open chamber instruments was the Evaporimeter (Servomed), which is nowadays replaced by the other two commercial devices claimed to be more accurate [10,13]: the Tewameter® TM 300 (Courage + Khazaka Electronic GmbH) and the Dermalab® equipped with a TEWL probe (Cortex Technology). The measuring chamber is approximately 2 cm high and 1 cm in diameter for both instruments.

Each humidity sensor is coupled or integrated in the same chip with a temperature sensor to compensate the oscillations in the RH measurements due to temperature fluctuations. Dermalab is not, strictly speaking, an open chamber instrument because its diffusion resistance is altered by the presence of a membrane in the top outlet, probably used to protect the sensors from air convection. Dermalab works in the range 0–250 $g/(m^2{\cdot}h)$ with a resolution of 0.1 $g/(m^2{\cdot}h)$. R is directly proportional to the chamber length and diameter. For the given dimensions, if the path in the chamber is not obstructed, R can be approximated to 990 $s{\cdot}m^{-1}$. For open chamber instruments, the measurement time typically ranges between 30 [5] and 45 s [14]. This delay is proportional to the time needed for the chamber to reach the same temperature of the skin. In the Tewameter 300, the probe is pre-heated to the range of skin temperature, 28–32°C, to obtain a stable measurement in about 15 s, which improves almost 50% the instrument response speed.

Nilsson also studied the effect of contact pressure between the probe and the skin surface. Stretching and compression of the skin due to the application of an excessive force may induce a variation of permeability and modify the optimal distance between the skin and the humidity sensors. He observed an increase of approximately 10% in the evaporation rate per 100 g of applied load and suggested not to

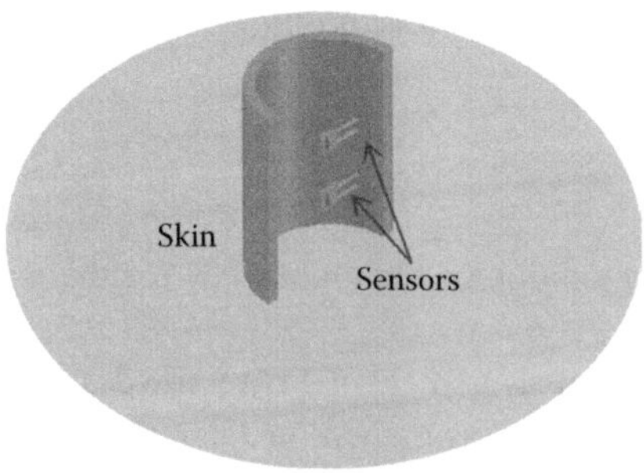

FIGURE 4.2 Cross-section of the cylindrical capsule with the humidity/temperature sensors used in the open chamber method.

exceed 40 g. On the other side, a weak contact with the skin can result in a vapor flow leakage. While the main advantage of the open chamber is that it allows for continuous measurements, the main drawback is the susceptibility to disturbances caused by air convection [15], e.g., air conditioning or breathing, and body-induced air currents [12]. Guidelines warn to place the instrument probe only on horizontal surfaces to avoid perturbations in the microclimate inside the chamber. Some authors suggest minimizing the impact of drafts by means of a shield protecting the open chamber [5,10]. However, this solution can be impractical and nearly resembles a closed chamber method, which is explained in the next section.

4.2.3 Closed Chamber

Another class of TEWL devices is based on a closed chamber approach. These devices are mainly divided into two categories, namely the *unventilated chamber* and the *condenser chamber*. Other closed chamber methods, currently not used in any commercial device, are discussed in Section 4.2.6.

4.2.4 Unventilated Chamber

Errors caused by air convection and body-induced air currents on the open chamber microclimate are particularly relevant at high evaporation rates because TEWL is underestimated. In addition, as discussed earlier, before the introduction of the probe heater in the Tewameter, measurement time was longer than 30 s to allow for TEWL stabilization. The first attempt to overcome these constraints was the development of the unventilated chamber method. Like in the open chamber, a capsule is placed on the skin, but the top side is closed. The water vapor loss is thus confined in the capsule and a single sensor measures the increase of humidity in the chamber (Figure 4.3).

The TEWL value is available in less than about 15 s. This measurement time is required to minimize the blocking effect of the chamber on the normal evaporation from skin. The first unventilated chamber-based instrument was the VapoMeter® (Delfintech Technologies Ltd.) [16]. It weighs 150 g and has a contact area of 1 cm^2. With the standard adapter, VapoMeter is claimed with a measurement time from 7 to

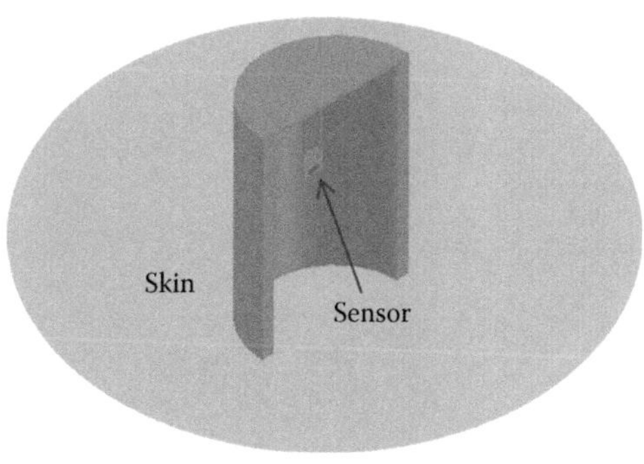

FIGURE 4.3 Cross-section of the probe used in the closed unventilated chamber approach.

15 s (10 s at the level of 10 g/(m²·h) and 16 s at 1 g/(m²·h)) and a TEWL measurement range from 3 to 200 g/(m²·h).

The rapid humidity increase in the capsule can be approximated by the following linear equation:

$$RH(t) = RH_a + kt \tag{4.5}$$

where t is the time, RH_a is the relative humidity of the capsule (equal to ambient RH) at $t = 0$, and k is the slope of the RH curve. The measurement usually starts after 3 to 4 seconds after the instrument is placed on the skin to skip the initial plateau of humidity. When humidity starts rising, the curve can be supposed linear and the measurement of the slope starts. It only lasts for a few seconds to avoid entering in the region of non-linearity. The mass of water m can be written as

$$m(t) = m_a + \Delta m \cdot t \cdot A \tag{4.6}$$

where m_a is the initial mass of water and A the surface area of evaporation. The change in mass Δm is the TEWL and is directly proportional to the slope k, which is calculated through a least square approximation. The proportionality constant can be calculated by a calibration procedure as described in [16]. Figure 4.4 shows an example of the rise of humidity and the time interval where the slope is evaluated.

Table 4.1 summarizes the updates to TEWL measurement guidelines [15] and indicates the preferred method, i.e., open or closed chamber, for different skin surface geometries and ranges of interest.

The performances of the VapoMeter are analyzed in a study conducted in [17] where the instrument is compared to Tewameter TM 210. Results show a good agreement between both systems, although the Tewameter measures higher values, probably because the VapoMeter calculates an average value whereas the Tewameter output is only available when the steady state is achieved. Tewameter seems more

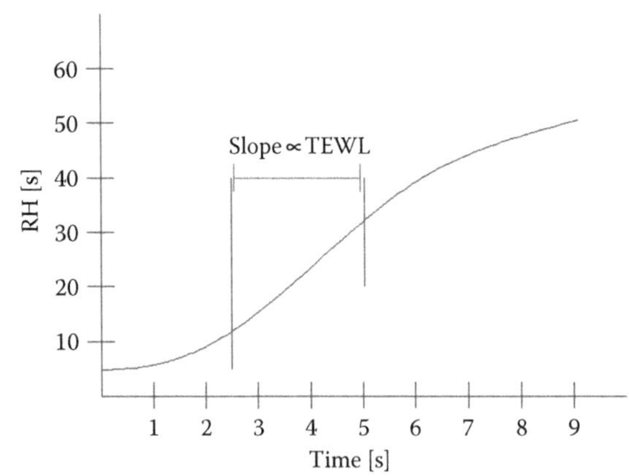

FIGURE 4.4 Example of the change of humidity in time. TEWL is proportional to the slope of the curve segment where linearity can be assumed.

TABLE 4.1
Preferred Methods for TEWL Measurements According to Skin Surface Geometry or Ranges of Interest

Measurement Method	Skin Surface Geometry	Range [g/(m2·h)]
Open or closed chamber	Flat	5–20
Closed chamber*	Curved	20–80
Closed chamber**	Area of diameter < 8 mm	80–200

* With short measurement time.
** With very short measurement time.
Source: J. Nuutinen, "Measurement of Transepidermal Water Loss by Closed-Chamber Systems," in *Handbook of Non-Invasive Methods and the Skin*, Second Ed., J. Serup, G.B.E. Jemec, G. Grove, Boca Raton: CRC Press, 2006, pp. 411–420.

precise at low TEWL values, which can be explained by the fact that when the slope change is small, the VapoMeter cannot correctly discriminates between the initial plateau and the increase in RH. The VapoMeter probe is found to be very sensitive to temperature variations when held with both hands, therefore the operator should take the necessary precautions to handle it.

The unventilated chamber method, and in general the closed chamber, seem to be less prone to disturbances due to the angle of measurement, but there is still some debate whether this is true. An advantage of the VapoMeter is the portability, as the entire instrument is hand-held because of its limited dimensions, 175 × 40 × 35 mm, and weight. In the last version, a wireless connection is available to retrieve data automatically from a personal computer. However, there are also some limitations, namely (a) the impossibility to perform continuous measurements because the water vapor needs to be purged off from the chamber after each measurement, which is an operation that takes longer time at higher evaporation rate; (b) the sensitivity to tremor and skin movements [18].

Another instrument inspired by the unventilated chamber method is the H4300 (Nikkiso-Ysi Co.) [19]. The H4300 is portable, but is not as small and light as the VapoMeter. The probe is equipped with 1.8 cm high – 0.8 cm in diameter capsule. TEWL value is ready after 18 s and the purging time is 20 s. The calibration procedure is not known, but the results are in good correlation to those obtained by the Dermalab.

4.2.5 Condenser Chamber

Similarly to the unventilated chamber, the condenser chamber is closed at the top, but in this case the closure is a temperature-controlled condenser [20] set below the freezing point of water. The first commercial device based on the condenser chamber method is the AquaFlux (Biox Systems Ltd.). A schematic design is shown in Figure 4.5. The chamber is open at the bottom, which is the part in contact with the skin. The probe diameter is 3 mm and the diffusion resistance is 900 $s{\cdot}m^{-1}$. The

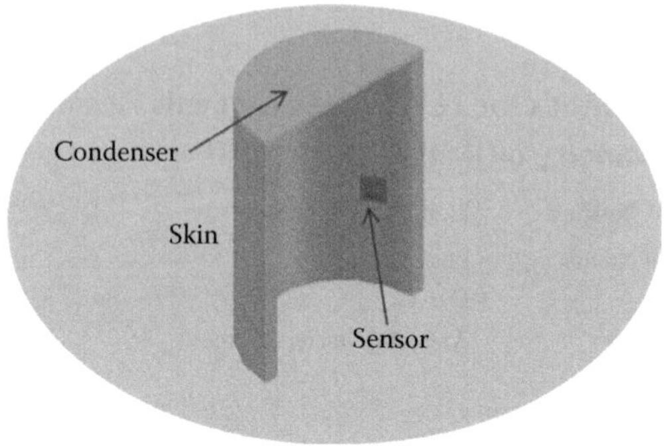

FIGURE 4.5 Cross-section of a condenser chamber TEWL sensor. The condenser is an aluminium plate controlled by a Peltier cooler and a heat sink.

condenser is an aluminum plate connected to a temperature controller composed of a Peltier cooler and a heat sink. A humidity sensor, coupled or integrated with a temperature sensor, is in the center of the chamber. AquaFlux AF200 can measure TEWL up to 250 g/(m^2·h).

The condenser chamber method can be described by a one-dimensional model, i.e., along the z-axis parallel to the chamber, if the following assumptions are true: (1) the capsule is adiabatic or, at least, the contribution to thermal conductivity is negligible; (2) the capsule wall has a low water affinity. A further hypothesis is to assume the internal dimensions of the capsule to be small enough to neglect any bulk air movement. Given the skin surface at position $z = 0$, the condenser at $z = L_c$, and the RH/T sensor at $z = L_s$, for a steady state water vapor flow, i.e., J = constant in Equation (4.2), the water evaporated at $z = 0$ is purged off by the condenser at $z = L_c$. The flow can be written as

$$J = D\left(\frac{\rho_s - \rho_c}{L_c - L_s}\right) \tag{4.7}$$

where ρ_s and ρ_c are the vapor densities at z equal to L_s and L_c, respectively. The vapor density can be written as

$$\rho = \chi \cdot \rho_E(T) \tag{4.8}$$

where χ is the fractional RH and ρ_E is the saturation vapor density. Therefore, since χ at $z = L_c$ is equal to 1, substituting Equation (4.8) in Equation (4.7) we have

$$J = \frac{D}{L_c - L_s}[\chi_S \rho_E(T_s) - \rho_E(T_c)] \tag{4.9}$$

where T_S and T_c are the temperatures at $z = L_s$ and $z = L_c$, respectively. Hence, the vapor flow can be calculated from χ_S, T_S and T_c. From Equation (4.9), substituting with $z = 0$, it follows that the relative humidity at the skin surface is

$$\chi_0 = \frac{\rho_E(T_s) + \left(J \cdot \frac{L_c}{D}\right)}{\rho_E(T_0)} \tag{4.10}$$

The main advantage of the condenser chamber method is the control of the microclimate humidity inside the chamber independently of external humidity. The humidity at the condenser is stable and does not change over time.

A recent *in vivo* study compares the condenser-chamber (AquaFlux AF200), the unventilated-chamber (VapoMeter SWL-2), and the open-chamber systems (Tewameter TM210) [21]. The authors' conclusion is that the measurements performed with the three instruments are significantly correlated although the condenser-chamber method should overcome the limitations of the VapoMeter and Tewameter, i.e., the tendency to skin occlusion resulting in a change in the microclimate close to the skin and sensitivity to air convection. However, the reported readings were at relative low values of TEWL. AquaFlux developers claim that their instrument is more precise at higher TEWL values, as it has a higher saturation detection limit, i.e., the flux density at which the air immediately adjacent to the skin surface is at 100% RH. An advantage over the closed chamber is that the condenser chamber method allows for many consecutive measurements, even though non-indefinitely like in the open chamber method. The condenser removes the water vapor by turning it into ice that accumulates on the aluminum surface. For the model AquaFlux AF200, authors report a decrease in sensitivity of about 1% every 2.5 mg of ice, which is equivalent to 500 continuous measurements at TEWL of 10 $g/(m^2 \cdot h)$ on the volar forearm.

4.2.6 Other Closed Chamber Methods

Literature reports at least two other TEWL measurement techniques based on the unventilated chamber principle. These methods are among the first attempts to measure TEWL and, despite being far surpassed in sensitivity and reliability, they are worth mentioning.

Electrical hygrometry was a rapid system to determine the relative humidity in a specific environment. In [22], it is described as a hygrometer based on a plastic wafer where a graphite circuit is printed. When the wafer adsorbs water molecules on the plastic surface, the electrical resistance of the graphite decreases. The hygrometer, which is calibrated to return the RH value, is suspended in a copper chamber with a thermocouple air thermometer.

An alternative is the gravimetric measurement of the water vapor content in a hygroscopic salt. In [23], authors try to assess the state of dermatitis in patients treated with corticosteroid drugs. They found evidence that TEWL reduction was associated with an improvement in the dermatitis condition. The sensing element is lithium chloride, i.e., a hygroscopic salt that varies its weight after absorbing water vapor. After calibration, the weight can be related to the amount of relative humidity in the closed chamber.

4.3 VENTILATED CHAMBER METHOD

The ventilated chamber method belongs to the earlier techniques to measure TEWL, like those described in Section 4.2.6. The evaporation rate is measured through a gas, e.g., nitrogen, continuously passed in the chamber (Figure 4.6). The speed and the water content of the gas are predefined.

TEWL is proportional to the product of the variation of vapor pressure between the incoming and outgoing gas and the gas speed. The amount of water vapor evaporated from the skin and captured by the gas can be evaluated by different approaches. Spruit [24] proposes a thermal conductivity cell housed in a container at 30°C. The system uses two thermistors, part of a Wheatstone bridge, to measure the difference in air temperature (a) entering in the cell and (b) after exchange with the water evaporated from the skin. Shahidullah et al. [25] described an unventilated chamber where the water vapor content in dry nitrogen was measured by electrolysis after absorption by phosphorus pentoxide. Other methods are based on gravimetric analysis [26] or infrared absorption [27].

Continuous measurements of TEWL are possible with the ventilated chamber method, but the sensitivity is low, especially for low water vapor content. The main drawback is the dependence on the gas speed that prevents a direct comparison of results unless they are related to speed zero.

4.4 HUMIDITY SENSORS

Although there are optical, gravimetric, piezoresistive, magnetoelastic humidity sensors [28], the most popular are resistive and capacitive [29]. The resistive sensor relies upon the change in conductivity when the sensing material adsorbs water molecules, whereas the capacitive RH sensor responds to the changes in the dielectric constant of the capacitor induced by the vapor uptake. The market offers several types of RH sensors, mainly based on ceramic materials, semiconductors, and polymers [30].

Typical ceramic compounds are Al_2O_3, TiO_2, and SiO_2. Al_2O_3 is widespread because of the high sensitivity to low content of water vapor due to its porosity, negligible variations on temperature changes, and the relative low manufacturing cost. Dielectric

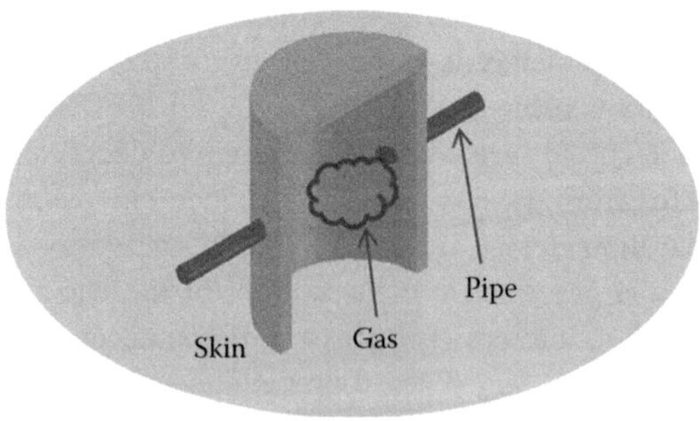

FIGURE 4.6 Cross-section of a ventilated chamber. A gas like nitrogen is continuously passed in the chamber. TEWL is proportional to the pressure difference at the pipe inlet and outlet times the gas speed.

α-Al_2O_3 films show the best performances in long-term stability (>1 year) and fast response (<5 s). An effective fabrication technique is reactive evaporation. A detection limit as low as 1 ppmv for the water vapor content has been achieved [31]. The use of TiO_2 as sensing material is twofold. Its intrinsic properties allow exploiting it as a semiconductor, both n- and p-type, as either a resistor or capacitor. Apart from some research works, TiO_2 is suitable for detecting humidity values in a small range, i.e., 10–30 RH%. Compared to Al_2O_3 and TiO_2, SiO_2 is less porous, but has the main advantage that the same fabrication process derived from the integrated circuits (IC) micro- and nanotechnology can be used for low cost mass production of humidity sensors.

Other sensing materials belong to the class of semiconductors such as SnO_2, ZnO, and In_2O_3 [30], carbon nitride [32], organic films [33], and metal phthalocyanines [34]. When water molecules are adsorbed on an n-type (p-type) semiconductor surface, an increase (decrease) in conductivity is observed. At room temperature, semiconductor humidity sensors usually exhibit longer response and recovery time than ceramics, but can easily be processed on a large scale.

Humidity sensors extensively employ polymer films for their high sensitivity, long stability, and low cost. Examples of resistive-type polymers are ammonium and sulfonate salts, Nafion™, polyvinyl alcohol (PVA), and polymethyl methacrylate (PMMA) [35]. PVA and PMMA are also known for their dielectric properties in capacitive humidity sensors. Other dielectric materials are cellulose acetate butyrate (CAB), polyimide (PI), vinyl methacrylate, and vinyl cinnamate [36].

4.5 ADVANCES IN TRANSEPIDERMAL WATER LOSS SENSORS

The commercial instruments above are the ones most widely used and constitute a *de facto* standard for TEWL measurement. In fact, because of their reliability and accurate results, at least when the operator correctly follows the recommendations described in the guidelines, they have reached a dominant position in the market. Nonetheless, the recent trend is to have wearable wireless sensors that, without external intervention, constantly monitor the user during his daily activity. None of the available instruments corresponds to this profile.

Publications and recent advances in technology usually focus on sweat detection and analysis, but the same achievements can often be extended to the study of TEWL. Salvo et al. [37] developed a prototype of a wearable sweat rate sensor that is a different application of the open chamber method. The sensor consists of two capacitive humidity sensors supported by two fabric nets held in place by a rubber gasket (Figure 4.7). The sensor is compared to VapoMeter during a 25 min cycling test. There is a good agreement between the two devices with the wearable sensor capable of following the VapoMeter curve in the recovery phase, i.e., when the user stops cycling, as well.

Other technological solutions show a methodology that is a point break with the chamber methods. A new generation of textiles, reasonably defined *smart* or *electronic*, is under test to start up a new class of fully wearable sensors capable of monitoring physiological parameters. These textiles require conductive elements to be embedded in the fabric. An option is to weave electrical components in a garment,

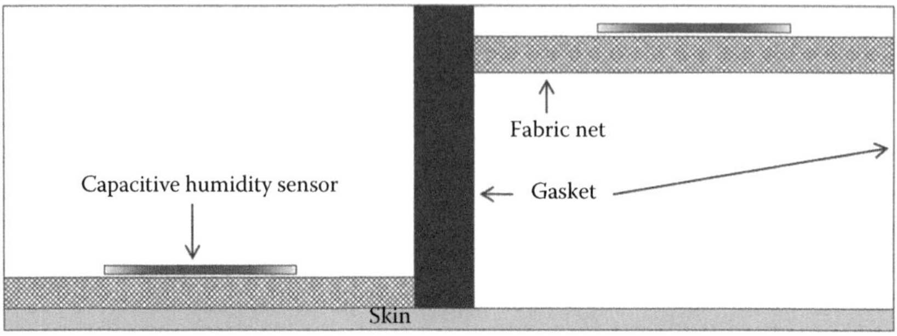

FIGURE 4.7 Cross-section of the wearable sweat rate sensor described in Salvo et al. [37]. The first humidity sensor is at a distance of 0.2 cm from the skin, while the second is 1 cm from the skin. The gasket is attached to the skin by a thin gel layer in order to reduce any noise due to body movements.

while the alternative is the fabrication of conductive fibers or yarns, which is the ultimate goal of wearable textiles. A potential TEWL sensor might derive from an organic electrochemical transistor (OECT). In [38], researchers have fabricated an organic field effect transistor where (a) the source and drain are on a cotton fiber functionalized with poly(3,4-ethylenedioxythiophene) doped with poly(styrene sulfonate) (PEDOT:PSS) conductive polymer; (b) the gate is a silver wire. The OECT has been successfully tested to detect the concentration of a NaCl solution simulating the human sweat. The OECT can directly work in liquid with less than 1 V supply. The density of charge carriers between the source and drain is modulated via capacitive coupling between the gate and the transistor channel, i.e., the functionalized cotton fiber. When the Na^+ and Cl^- accumulate between the Ag wire and the fiber, the charge density changes and modulates the OECT impedance. Therefore, the variation in the drain-source current provides a measurement of the concentration of ions in the transistor. This smart textile might be turned into a TEWL sensor working on the integration of similar humidity field effect organic transistors in fibers [39,40].

An interesting approach relies on the combination of a skin patch and a radio frequency identification (RFID) device [41]. The absorbent layer of the skin patch is made of a cellulose layer firmly held on the skin by a protective polyurethane layer, normally used as wound dressing (Tegaderm™ by 3M™). An additional film layer serves as a protective layer between the RFID coil and the cellulose layer. Tegaderm allows the patch to be breathable, thus preventing saturation by accumulation of water vapor, and at the same time blocks external molecules to enter in contact with the skin. At 1 KHz, the dielectric constant of polyurethane and cellulose are 3.2 and 3.85, respectively. When water vapor condenses on the RIFD coils, the capacitance hugely changes due to the high difference in dielectric constants of water (80 at room temperature) and polyurethane/cellulose. The shift in the RFID nominal frequency is related to the amount of fluid on the antenna. Thus, this wireless sensor can be used to measure the local evaporation rate in real-time. A drawback is the need of a receiving device to detect the frequency shift. The author used a vector network analyzer (8753D by Hewlett Packard), whose price and dimensions are not compatible with a low-cost portable instrument.

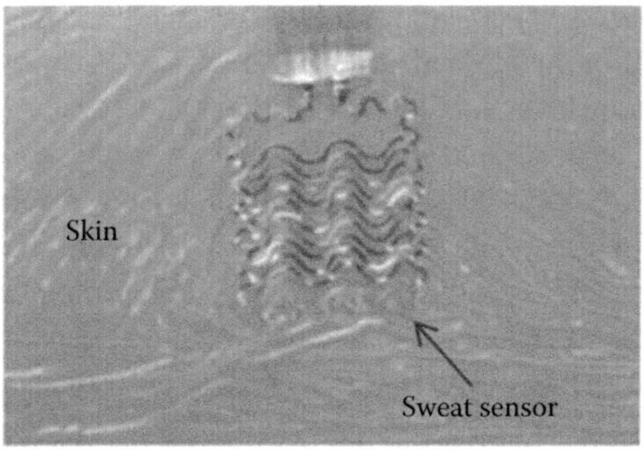

FIGURE 4.8 Stretchable, ultrathin, and conformable skin-mounted sweat rate sensor. (From Hsu, Y.Y. et al. "Epidermal Electronics: Skin Sweat Patch," in *7th International Microsystems, Packaging, Assembly and Circuits Technology Conference [IMPACT]*, Taipei, 2012. With permission.)

One of the most promising and interesting research projects is epidermal electronics [42], which are the new frontier of wearable sensors. This technology enables the fabrication of an ultrathin and stretchable system that can be laminated on the skin like a tattoo. Hsu et al. use this technique to develop a conformal skin patch sensitive to sweat level [43]. Previous works determine the sweat level by a set of electrodes that measure the impedance of the skin, but an excellent contact with the skin is necessary and the pressure applied on the electrodes influences the result. On the contrary, the epidermal circuit adapts to the skin surface without any external force to maintain the contact. The patch consists of a set of 100 μm wide and 0.5 μm thick interdigitated electrodes patterned by photolithography on a cellulose support. The top layer is a Tegaderm film that provides adhesion with the skin. Electrodes are made of gold encapsulated on a 10 μm thick layer of polyimide on both sides. The electrodes need to adapt their shape to the skin deformation minimizing the effects on their structural integrity. In fact, stretching causes cracks in the gold layer. As cracks propagate through the electrodes, the resistance increases. The classical rectangular shape is not adequate to sustain the stretches and it is substituted by a meander-like profile. The skin sweat patch is shown in Figure 4.8.

When cellulose absorbs the sweat, the resistivity starts decreasing because of the mobile ions present in sweat, mainly sodium, potassium, and chloride. Capacitance increases as explained for the above-mentioned RIFD patch. The authors demonstrate that the sensor has an operational limit equal to 40% of elongation. Above this threshold, both capacitance and impedance reach a saturation level, i.e., it is not possible to distinguish between different values of sweat rate.

4.6 CLOSING REMARKS

At present, the reliability and validity of TEWL measurements are only guaranteed by the commercial instruments based on the chamber methods, which undergo extensive tests by the scientific community. Articles on instruments validation and comparison are numerous and published in peer review journals. Cosmetics, dermatology, or sport science laboratories that need to assess TEWL can only choose among the aforementioned products because there is no valid alternative. New devices are under investigation, but neither the materials nor the methods are mature enough for accurate and repeatable tests. Prototypes are fragile and limited to research use. Nonetheless, the outlook for new devices is optimistic since pervasive wearable wireless sensors are the actual strategy for the development of new technologies that can extend the monitoring of physiological parameters outside controlled laboratories. Probably, the new technological generation will also lead to cost reduction, since current TEWL sensors cost several thousand euros.

REFERENCES

1. C. Rosado, P. Pinto, and L.M. Rodrigues, "Comparative assessment of the performance of two generations of Tewameter," *International Journal of Cosmetic Science*, vol. 27, no. 4, p. 237–241, 2005.
2. S.B. Hoath, "Physiologic Development of the Skin," in *Fetal and Neonatal Physiology*, Fourth Ed., vol. 1, Philadelphia: Elsevier Saunders, 2011, pp. 679–695.
3. L. Talakoub, I.M. Neuhaus, and S.S. Yu, "Cosmeceuticals," in *Cosmetic Dermatology: Requisites in Dermatology Series*, Second Ed., M. Alam, H.B. Gladstone, and R.C. Tung, eds., Philadelphia: Elsevier Saunders, 2009, pp. 7–34.
4. L.O. Lamke, G.E. Nilsson, and H.L. Reithner, "The evaporative water loss from burns and the water-vapor permeability of grafts and artificial membranes used in the treatment of burns," *Burns*, vol. 3, no. 3, pp. 159–165, 1977.
5. J. du Plessis, A. Stefaniak, F. Eloff, S. John, T. Agner, T.C. Chou, R. Nixon, M. Steiner, A. Franken, I. Kudla, and L. Holness, "International guidelines for the *in vivo* assessment of skin properties in non-clinical settings: Part 2. Transepidermal water loss and skin hydration," *Skin Research and Technology*, vol. In press, 2013.
6. A. Patzelt, W. Sterry, and J. Lademann, "*In vivo* measurements of skin barrier: Comparison of different methods and advantages of laser scanning microscopy," *Laser Physics Letters*, vol. 7, no. 12, pp. 843–852, 2010.
7. G.E. Nilsson, "Measurement of water exchange through skin," *Medical and Biological Engineering and Computing*, vol. 15, no. 3, pp. 209–218, 1977.
8. R.C. Roberts, "Diffusion of Gases," in *American Institute of Physics Handbook*, New York: McGraw-Hill, 1957, pp. 211–214.
9. C. Antoine, "Tensions des vapeurs: Nouvelle relation entre les tensions et les températures," *Comptes Rendus des Séances de l'Académie des Sciences*, vol. 107, pp. 681–684, 778–780, 836–837, 1888.
10. R.E. Imhof, M.E.P. De Jesus, P. Xiao, L.I. Ciortea, and E.P. Berg, "Closed-chamber transepidermal water loss measurement: Microclimate, calibration and performance," *International Journal of Cosmetic Science*, vol. 31, pp. 97–118, 2009.
11. V. Rogiers and EEMCO Group, "EEMCO guidance for the assessment of transepidermal water loss in cosmetic sciences," *Skin Pharmacology and Applied Skin Physiology*, vol. 14, no. 2, pp. 117–128, 2001.
12. J. Pinnagoda, R.A. Tupker, T. Agner, and J. Serup, "Guidelines for transepidermal water loss (TEWL) measurement. A report from the Standardization Group of the European Society of Contact Dermatitis," *Contact Dermatitis*, vol. 22, pp. 164–178, 1990.
13. G.L. Grove, M.J. Grove, C. Zerweck, and E. Pierce, "Comparative metrology of the evaporimeter and the DermaLab TEWL probe," *Skin Research and Technology*, vol. 5, pp. 1–8, 1999.

14. J. Pinnagoda, R.A. Tupker, P.J. Coenraads, and J.P. Nater, "Comparability and Reproducibility of Results of Water Vapor Loss Measurements: A Study of Four Evaporimeters," in *Current Topics in Contact Dermatitis*, P. Frosch, A. Dooms-Goossens, J. Lachapelle, R.J.G. Rycroft, and J. Scheper, eds., New York: Springer, 1989, pp. 560–564.
15. J. Nuutinen, "Measurement of Transepidermal Water Loss by Closed-Chamber Systems," in *Handbook of Non-Invasive Methods and the Skin*, Second Ed., J. Serup, G.B.E. Jemec, G. Grove, Boca Raton: CRC Press, 2006, pp. 411–420.
16. J. Nuutinen, E. Alanen, P. Autio, M.R. Lahtinen, I. Harvima, and T. Lahtinen, "A closed unventilated chamber for the measurement of transepidermal water loss," *Skin Research and Technology*, vol. 9, pp. 85–89, 2003.
17. K. De Paepe, E. Houben, R. Adam, F. Wiesemann, and V. Rogiers, "Validation of the VapoMeter, a closed unventilated chamber system to assess transepidermal water loss vs. the open chamber Tewameter," *Skin Research and Technology*, vol. 11, pp. 61–69, 2005.
18. E. Alanen, F. Wiesemann, J. Nuutinen, and T. Lahtinen, "Measurement of skin hydration in the diapered area of infants with a closed chamber TEWL meter," *Skin Research and Technology*, vol. 9, no. 2, pp. 199–200, 2003.
19. H. Tagami, H. Kobayashi, and K. Kikuchi, "A portable device using a closed chamber system for measuring transepidermal water loss: Comparison with the conventional method," *Skin Research and Technology*, vol. 8, no. 1, pp. 7–12, 2002.
20. R.E. Imhof, E.P. Berg, R.P. Chilcott, L.I. Ciortea, and F.C. Pascut, "New instrument for measuring water vapor flux density from arbitrary surfaces," *IFSCC Magazine*, vol. 5, no. 4, pp. 297–301, 2002.
21. S. Farahmand, L. Tien, X. Hui, and H.I. Maibach, "Measuring transepidermal water loss: A comparative *in vivo* study of condenser-chamber, unventilated-chamber and open-chamber systems," *Skin Research and Technology*, vol. 15, pp. 392–398, 2009.
22. E.W. Rosenberg, H. Blank, and S. Resnik, "Sweating and water loss through the skin," *JAMA*, vol. 179, no. 10, pp. 809–811, 1962.
23. M. Shahidullah, E.J. Raffle, and W. Frain-Bell, "Insensible water loss in dermatitis," *British Journal of Dermatology*, vol. 79, no. 11, pp. 589–597, 1967.
24. D. Spruit, "Measurement of the water vapor loss from human skin by a thermal conductivity cell," *Journal of Applied Physiology*, vol. 23, no. 6, pp. 994–997, 1967.
25. M. Shahidullah, E.J. Raffle, A.R. Rimmer, and W. Frain-Bell, "Transepidermal water loss in patient with dermatitis," *British Journal of Dermatology*, vol. 81, pp. 722–730, 1969.
26. G.E. Burch and T. Windsor, "Rate of insensible perspiration (diffusion of water) locally through living and through dead human skin," *Archives of Internal Medicine*, vol. 74, no. 6, pp. 437–444, 1944.
27. C. Johnson and S. Shuster, "The measurement of transepidermal water loss," *British Journal of Dermatology*, vol. 81, no. Supplement s4, pp. 40–46, 1969.
28. C.Y. Lee and G.B. Lee, "Humidity sensors: A review," *Sensor Letters*, vol. 3, no. 1–4, pp. 1–15, 2005.
29. P. Salvo, "Sweat Rate Wearable Sensors," in *Biological and Medical Sensor Technologies*, K. Iniewski, ed., Boca Raton: CRC Press, 2012, pp. 243–262.
30. Z. Chen and C. Lu, "Humidity sensors: A review of materials and mechanisms," *Sensor Letters*, vol. 3, pp. 274–295, 2005.
31. Z. Chen, M. Jin, and C. Zhen, "Humidity sensors with reactively evaporated Al2O3 films as porous dielectrics," *Sensors and Actuators B: Chemical*, vol. 2, no. 3, pp. 167–171, 1990.
32. S.P. Lee, J.G. Lee, and S. Chowdhury, "CMOS humidity sensor system using carbon nitride film as sensing materials," *Sensors*, vol. 8, pp. 2662–2672, 2008.

33. S.A. Moiz, M.M. Ahmed, and K.S. Karimov, "Effects of temperature and humidity on electrical properties of organic semiconductor orange dye films deposited from solution," *Japanese Journal of Applied Physics*, vol. 44, no. 3, pp. 1199–1203, 2005.
34. F. Aziz, M.H. Sayyad, K.S. Karimov, M. Saleem, Z. Ahmad, and S.M. Khan, "Characterization of vanadyl phthalocyanine based surface-type capacitive humidity sensors," *Journal of Semiconductors*, vol. 31, no. 11, pp. 114002-1-114002–6, 2010.
35. Z.M. Rittersma, "Recent achievements in miniaturised humidity sensors—A review of transduction techniques," *Sensors and Actuators A*: *Physical*, vol. 96, no. 2–3, pp. 196–210, 2002.
36. Y. Sakai, Y. Sadaoka, and M. Matsuguchi, "Humidity sensors based on polymer thin films," *Sensors and Actuators B*: *Chemical*, Vols. 35-36, pp. 85–90, 1996.
37. P. Salvo, F. Di Francesco, D. Costanzo, C. Ferrari, M.G. Trivella, and D. De Rossi, "A wearable sensor for measuring sweat rate," *IEEE Sensors Journal*, vol. 10, no. 10, pp. 1557–1558, 2010.
38. G. Tarabella, M. Villani, D. Calestani, R. Mosca, S. Iannotta, A. Zappettini, and N. Coppedè, "A single cotton fiber organic electrochemical transistor for liquid electrolyte saline sensing," *Journal of Materials Chemistry*, vol. 22, pp. 23830–23834, 2012.
39. L. Torsi, A. Dodabalapur, N. Cioffi, L. Sabbatini, and P.G. Zambonin, "NTCDA organic thin-film-transistor as humidity sensor: Weaknesses and strengths," *Sensors and Actuators B*: *Chemical*, vol. 77, no. 1–2, pp. 7–11, 2001.
40. S.P. Lee and K.J. Park, "Humidity sensitive field effect transistors," *Sensors and Actuators B*: *Chemical*, vol. 35, no. 1–3, pp. 80–84, 1996.
41. L.E. Klinker, "Skin-Based Sweat Monitoring Using Radio Frequency Identification Sensors," Tufts University, Honors Thesis, 2012.
42. D.-H. Kim, N. Lu, R. Ma, Y -S. Kim, R.-H. Kim, S. Wang, J. Wu, S. M. Won, H. Tao, A. Islam, K.J. Yu, T.I. Kim, R. Chowdhury, M. Ying, L. Xu, M. Li, H.J. Chung, H. Keum, M. McCormick, P. Liu, Y.-W. Zhang, F.G. Omenetto, Y. Huang, T. Coleman, and J.A. Rogers, "Epidermal electronics," *Science*, vol. 333, pp. 838–843, 2011.
43. Y.Y. Hsu, J. Hoffman, R. Ghaffari, B. Ives, P. Wei, L. Klinker, B. Morey, B. Elolampi, D. Davis, C. Rafferty, and K. Dowling, "Epidermal Electronics: Skin Sweat Patch," in 7th International Microsystems, Packaging, Assembly and Circuits Technology Conference (IMPACT), Taipei, 2012.

5 Portable High-Frequency Ultrasound Imaging System Design and Hardware Considerations*

Insoo Kim, Hyunsoo Kim, Flavio Griggio, Richard L. Tutwiler, Thomas N. Jackson, Susan Trolier-McKinstry, and Kyusun Choi

CONTENTS

* Previously published in Iniewski, K., ed. (2011) *Integrated Microsystems: Electronics, Photonics, and Biotechnology,* Boca Raton, FL: CRC Press.

5.1 INTRODUCTION

Ultrasound techniques have wide use in various applications in numerous fields. The frequency range from 10 KHz to 1 MHz is widely used for SONAR (sound navigation and ranging), ultrasonic welding, therapeutic ultrasound, and humidifiers. A frequency range of 1–50 MHz is common in diagnostic sonography and nondestructive testing to find flaws in materials. Micron-sized silicon surface detection utilizes a frequency range of 50–200 MHz [1], and SAW (surface acoustic wave) devices use frequencies ranging from 1 to 10 GHz.

Ultrasound techniques are also common for diagnostic imaging and often supersede x-ray imaging in the medical sector [2]. The vast majority of medical ultrasound imaging occurs at frequencies between 1 and 50 MHz. For example, diagnostic imaging designed to penetrate tissues to a depth of 5–20 cm uses frequencies between 1 and 10 MHz. Recently, studies for imaging smaller organs or surfaces, such as skin, the gastrointestinal tract, and intravascular blood vessels, have emerged utilizing ultrasound with frequencies over 20 MHz. However, a need remains for better clinical ultrasound imaging for detecting skin, eye, and prostate cancers as well as many other diseases, *in vivo*. Imaging techniques with a resolution below 100 μm for these situations would minimize the need for biopsies [2].

Moreover, the medical community has recently expressed a desire for an ultrasound imaging system that would not only provide appropriate resolution but also would be portable [3]. For example, veterinarians would be well served by development of a portable ultrasound imaging system for onsite diagnosis of pets, and zoo and farm animals. The conventional system's size is due to the complex front-end electronics that consist of discrete chipsets for pulsers, preamplifiers, TGCs (time gain controls), A/D (analog/digital) converters, and memory devices. In addition, the conventional design of the transducer arrays requires high-transmit-drive voltages on the order of 100 V.

During the past 20 years or so, many researchers have tried to produce miniaturized and integrated ultrasound imaging systems [4–10]. It is because integrating all electronic components into a single IC chip affords a smaller system size, higher speed, and lower power consumption than building the system with discrete chipsets. The early ultrasound ASIC chips were reported by Black et al. and Hatfield et al. in

1994. The ASIC chips contained 16 channels of transmitters and current amplifiers with integrated transducers [4] and digital transmitters [5]. Since 2000, with the rapid development of mixed-signal IC design technology, closed-coupled ultrasound front-end electronics have emerged for high-frequency ultrasound imaging systems. Wygant et al. developed a CMUT (capacitive micromachined ultrasound transducer) with closed-coupled electronics [6], which contain 16 receive-transmit channels. Johansson et al. introduced a portable ultrasound system using a battery-operated voltage-boosting scheme [7]. The Sonic Window, developed by Fuller et al. in 2005, included one of the most integrated ultrasound front-end IC chip concepts to date [8]. Developed for guiding needle and catheter insertion, biopsies, and other invasive procedures for which only a basic aid to diagnosis is necessary, the Sonic Window can also be used for C-mode ultrasound imaging.

Kim et al. introduced a high-frequency system with a fully integrated, custom-designed ultrasound front-end IC chip, which includes both transmit and receive electronics with A/D converters and high-capacity on-chip memory [9]. The design has integrated electronics with thin-film transducers small enough to construct a portable, ultra-compact, low-power consumption ultrasound imaging system. Unlike other works mentioned earlier, which still require a significantly higher drive voltage for excitation of transducers, the transceiver chip interfaces with thin-film transducer arrays that operate below 5 V, so that the limitations of high-voltage excitation become moot.

This chapter focuses on introducing the architecture and design of a fully integrated ultrasound transceiver chip. Section 5.2 outlines the key points of ultrasound imaging fundamentals: ultrasound physics, the basics of B-mode ultrasound imaging, and beamforming architectures. Section 5.3 investigates the design consideration for ultrasound transceiver chip in portable high-frequency ultrasound imaging systems. Section 5.4 presents the Penn State portable ultrasound imaging system. The design specifications and details of the circuit components on the transceiver chip are described. In addition, the characteristics of the transceiver chip and measured signal acquisition results from the Penn State ultrasound imaging system along with the thin-film ultrasound transducer arrays are shown. Last, the summary and the conclusions are addressed in Section 5.5.

5.2 B-MODE ULTRASOUND IMAGING SYSTEM

5.2.1 Ultrasound Imaging Basics

An ultrasound wave is a longitudinal wave in which oscillations are in the same direction as propagation. In addition, the ultrasound wave is attenuated as it propagates through the medium. Several factors contribute to this attenuation. One of the most significant factors is the absorption of ultrasound energy by the medium and its conversion into heat. The ultrasound wave loses its acoustic energy continuously as it moves through the medium. Scattering and refraction also result in some loss of energy and contribute to overall attenuation.

Reflection is an important physical phenomenon of an ultrasound wave, and it is also a key characteristic used for ultrasound imaging. A reflection occurs at any boundary between two media having different densities and/or acoustic velocities.

When an ultrasound wave encounters the boundary between two media, only a portion of the wave's acoustic energy will be transmitted, and the rest of the acoustic energy will be reflected. B-mode ultrasound imaging is based on the pulse-echo (backscattering) response of an ultrasound wave, and provides a two-dimensional, cross-sectional reflection image of the scanned object [10]. The amplitude of reflection signal is converted to the brightness information of the target object. Higher amplitude creates a brighter image, and weaker amplitude creates a dark image.

In the meantime, the ultrasound wave is attenuated as it propagates through the medium. Several factors contribute to this attenuation. One of the most significant factors is the absorption of ultrasound energy by the medium and its conversion into heat. The ultrasound wave loses its acoustic energy continuously as it moves through the medium. Scattering and refraction also result in some loss of energy and contribute to overall attenuation. A simple exponential loss of pressure amplitude expresses the attenuation of an ultrasound wave [11]:

$$p(z) = p_0 e^{-\alpha(f)\times z} \tag{5.1}$$

where

p_0 is the initial pressure amplitude

$\alpha(f)$ is the attenuation coefficient that is a function of frequency

This implies that the reflection signal from the closer medium from the observation point is stronger than the reflection signals from the far medium even if the media are the same. Therefore, time-gain compensator (TGC) is necessary in the ultrasound front-end electronics to compensate for signal attenuation as a function of depth.

Resolution is one of the most important properties to consider in designing an ultrasound imaging system. Resolution involves two factors in a B-scan: (1) resolution in the direction of the transducer motion, known as "lateral" or "transverse" resolution, and (2) resolution in the direction of acoustic pulse propagation, known as "axial" resolution.

Lateral resolution of an ultrasound imaging system (resolution in the direction of transducer motion) is the system's ability to discriminate between two closely adjacent structures placed at the same depth from the transducer surface. The ultrasound's beam width at a specific depth determines lateral resolution. The beam width varies as the wave propagates in and out of the focal region; therefore, the focusing property of the transducer is

$$L.R. = f^{\#}\lambda = \frac{f}{a}\lambda \tag{5.2}$$

where

$f^{\#}$ is the *f*-number

a is the aperture of the transducer

f is a focal length

λ is a wavelength

Practically, lateral resolution is proportional to 2λ [12].

Axial resolution of an ultrasound imaging system (resolution in the direction of ultrasound wave propagation) is the ability to discriminate between two closely placed structures lying along the length of the ultrasound wave. The important factor in determining axial resolution is the spatial pulse length (λ) and the numbers of pulses (*N*)

$$A.R. = \frac{N\lambda}{2} \tag{5.3}$$

From both (5.2) and (5.3), notably, the wavelength, and consequently the frequency, directly determines the resolution of an ultrasound system. In general, a higher-frequency ultrasound wave is more desirable for higher resolution. However, arbitrarily increasing the ultrasound wave frequency to obtain finer resolution is not desirable because the attenuation rate of ultrasound waves increase as the frequency increases. Therefore, in determining frequency, a necessary consideration is the trade-off between the resolution and the penetration distance of the ultrasound wave. Having set the frequency of an ultrasound wave, the specification for the front-end electronics, such as input buffer bandwidth and A/D conversion speed, can be determined.

5.2.2 B-Mode Imaging System Hardware

A block diagram of a general B-mode ultrasound imaging system appears in Figure 5.1. The following subsections generically describe the processing blocks.

5.2.2.1 Control Host

This grouping includes microprocessors or a host computer and postprocessors. The computer or microprocessors control the entire hardware system to function in the desired modes and to provide a control interface to the front-end electronics. The post-processor performs scan conversions (i.e., imaging formation), image processing, and display.

5.2.2.2 T/R Switch

Generally, the transmit pulses use a very high voltage, typically up to 200 V, while the receiver electronics process lower voltages signals in the 10^{-3} volt range. Modern CMOS technology uses a power supply of below 5 V. Therefore, the receiver should be isolated from transmit pulses in order to protect inner circuits. The T/R switch

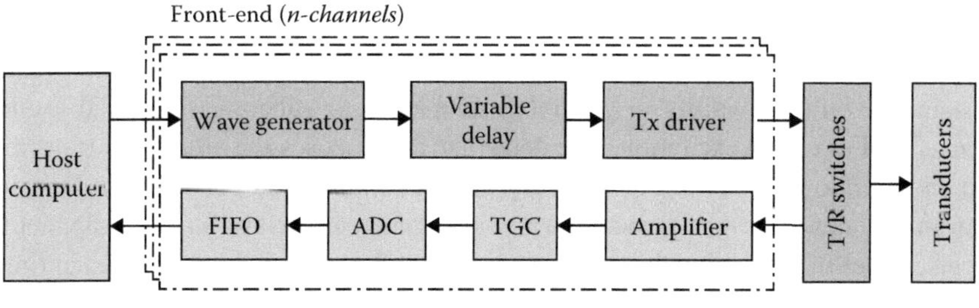

FIGURE 5.1 A block diagram of a general B-mode ultrasound imaging system.

connects transducers to the transmitter during transmit mode operation; conversely, the switch connects the transducer to the receiver during receive mode operation.

5.2.2.3 Amplifier

The amplifier is a key component in the ultrasound imaging system. It performs two functions: first, it receives the reflected signals from the transducers. This means that the dynamic range of the amplifier is crucial because attenuation of an ultrasound wave is sometimes over 100 dB. Impedance matching between the amplifier and the transducers is also important for reception. A low-noise amplifier (LNA), which has both high dynamic range and good impedance-matching properties, is preferred for the preamplifier. Second, the preamplifier enhances the received signals, but careful preamplifier gain selection avoids amplified signal saturation.

5.2.2.4 TGC

The TGC provides time-varying gain for the reflected ultrasound signal whose attenuation varies as a function of depth and the attenuation coefficient of the medium. From Equation (5.1), ultrasound waves attenuate on a logarithmic scale rather than a linear scale. This means that the TGC should express a variable linear gain range in the dB scale. The TGC can be a variable gain amplifier (VGA).

5.2.2.5 A/D Converter and Memory (FIFO)

Every receive channel needs one or more A/D converters for digital beamforming (DBF). The conversion rates of three to five times the highest center frequency are necessary to reduce beamforming quantization errors [13]. As conversion speed increases, memory devices may be needed to store the digitized data and to interface the A/D converter with the receive beamformer.

5.2.3 Beamforming

Modern ultrasound imaging systems often use multichannel transducer arrays to increase beam flexibility, spatial convergence, and resolution. Ultrasound pulses from each channel should have a delay in order to form a wave front that converges on a specified focal point. The transmit beamformer generates delays for each channel to focus and steer the transmit beam, and the receive beamformer performs focusing and steering of the scattered RF signals to create the B-mode images. In certain systems, the transmitter consists of delay networks. A single cycle pulse excitation signal is ideal for B-mode imaging since it yields better axial resolution. Typical systems have the flexibility to generate multiple-gated bursts of sinusoidal excitation as well as coded excitation. The delay network focuses the amount of transmitted energy into the medium and has capability for pulse and pulsed-wave Doppler transmit modes. The receive beamformer also generates delays for each channel in inverse order of transmit delays to align the amplified signals at the reference time. Then, the post-processor adds the delay compensated signals and generates a large imaging signal for further image processing.

5.2.3.1 Analog Beamforming versus Digital Beamforming

Beamforming architectures are of two types: analog beamforming (ABF) and DBF. ABF for ultrasound waves first appeared in the 1960s. Researchers developed DBF in the 1980s; however, not until the 1990s did DBF become feasible, because that period made available fast, high-precision A/D converters necessary for these systems. The recent development of very large-scale integration (VLSI) techniques enables designing real-time digital receive beamformers, and allows amplified signals from receive channels to be coherently added after digitization [14].

The main difference between ABF and DBF, as compared in Figure 5.2, is the method of achieving beamforming. In ABF, analog delay lines for each channel delay transmit pulses, then the beam is formed. In receive mode, the amplified and delayed, reflected analog signal compensates for the transmit delays, which are subsequently accumulated to construct a large analog imaging signal. Then, an ADC digitizes the analog signal for further image processing.

Unlike the signals in an ABF system, the signals in a DBF system are sampled as close to the transducer elements as possible in receive mode, and then delayed and summed digitally. Thus, a DBF system needs an A/D converter for each channel. Since modern DBF systems use multichannels and arrays of transducers, DBF

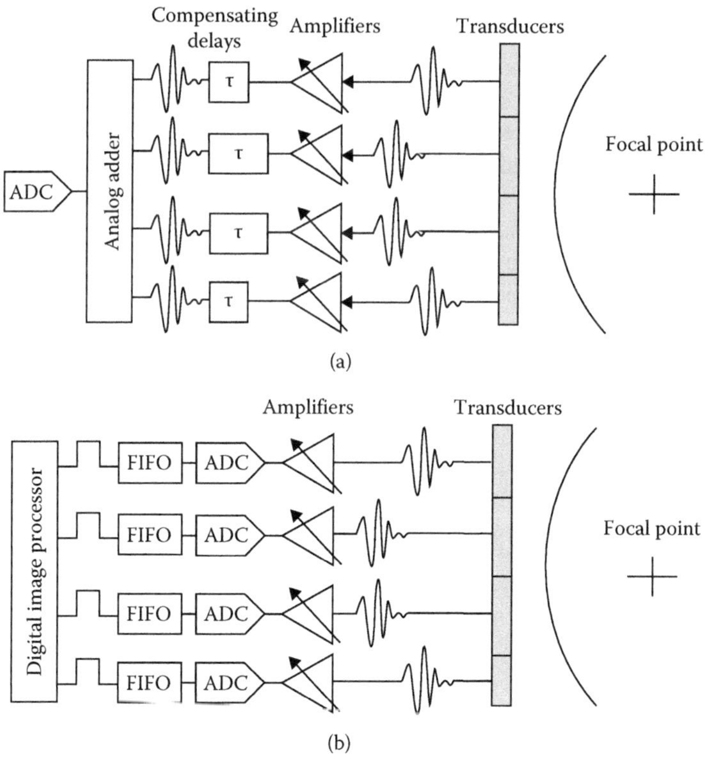

FIGURE 5.2 Simple block diagram of a typical DBF system: (a) receive analog beamforming system, (b) receive digital beamforming system.

requires a large number of A/D converters. This creates a considerable disadvantage for DBF systems since ADCs consume significant power.

However, DBF systems also have considerable advantages over ABF systems. First, DBF has better control over time-delay quantization errors. Analog delay lines tend to be poorly matched between channels. In DBF, synchronization with a high-frequency clock source can greatly improve delay accuracy. Second, DBF provides a finer resolution of ultrasound images. Typical analog delay accuracy is on the order of 20 ns, which constrains lateral resolution [12], but digital delay accuracy in modern digital circuit technology is on the order of a few hundred picoseconds with a few gigahertz clock sources and PLLs (phase locked loop) [15]. Last, since the digitized data is much less susceptible to noise than analog signal, DBF systems, in stark contrast to ABF systems, can deliver clearer display images than ABF systems, which may have analog noise throughout its entire system.

5.3 CHALLENGES TO PORTABLE HIGH-FREQUENCY ULTRASOUND IMAGING SYSTEMS

5.3.1 Low-Voltage High-Frequency Transducer

The majority of existing transducers for medical imaging still need a significantly higher drive voltage for excitation (above 60 V). High-voltage excitation pulses result in more complex system designs requiring protection T/R (Transmit/Receive) switches, digital controls, and charge-pump circuitry for the transmitter. Thus, the high voltage system is apt to consume high power, and consequently, is not suitable for portable systems. In addition, the existing systems interface the transducer array elements with the RF front-end by coaxial cable networks. The cables are specifically 50 ohm impedance matched to the RF front-end interface. The existence of T/R switches between the cable network and the front-end electronics makes impedance matching even more complex.

Therefore, low-voltage high-frequency ultrasound transducer arrays are crucial in portable high-frequency ultrasound imaging systems. The low-voltage transducers make the imaging system capable of integrating front-end electronics with transducers without charge-pump circuitry and RF coaxial cables. In addition, receiver protection devices are likely to be unnecessary because the transmit voltage is of the same magnitude as the CMOS logic voltage level. The integrated electronics also produces better signal integrity and noise immunity than conventional, analog, front-end electronics, which consist of discrete chipsets. Digital signal interfacing has wide acceptance for much higher signal-to-noise ratio (SNR) compliance than analog signal interfacing. In conventional systems, substantial efforts are necessary to control SNR in analog signal interfacing. However, in the integrated system, only chip-to-chip interfacing is necessary via digital signals because all analog signal processing occurs inside the chip and chips produce only digital outputs.

Researches on developing low-voltage high-frequency ultrasound transducers are in demand. First, the high-frequency PZT thin-film ultrasound transducer arrays using MEMS technology are proposed in [16]. The PZT layers can be thin, and allow reduction of the required voltages for exciting the transducer. The center frequency of the thin-film transducer is 30–70 MHz with a bandwidth of 60%–100%. Because the piezoelectric layer is a thin film (<1 μm thickness), the transducer array utilizes CMOS-compatible, low-level (below 5 V) excitation voltages. This technology enables the thin-film ultrasound transducers to be placed in close proximity to the electronics.

In addition, 20-element high-frequency ultrasound transducer array using micromolding technique is introduced in [17]. The array used piezocomposite material and thin-film Cr–Au electrodes in a mask-based process, packaged in epoxy with external connectors. The center frequency of the transducer is about 35 MHz with a bandwidth of 74% at 6 dB points.

5.3.2 Hardware Specifications

Achieving the required design specification for a high-frequency ultrasound imaging system is challenging. The linear dynamic range for an analog amplifier has a limitation of 100 dB in practical systems. However, the required dynamic range of the preamplifiers is sometimes higher than 100 dB for an ultrasound imaging system [3]. An even more critical obstacle is the requirements for the A/D converter. While the earliest commercially available digital beamformers became available in the early 1980s, they did not begin to have a significant impact until the early 1990s. Much of this delay was due to the need for A/D converters with sufficiently large numbers of bits and sufficiently high sampling rates.

Figure 5.3 shows the ADC development trends presented in the recent publications of two major international conferences: the ISSCC (International Solid State Circuits Conference) and the VLSI (Symposia on VLSI Technology and

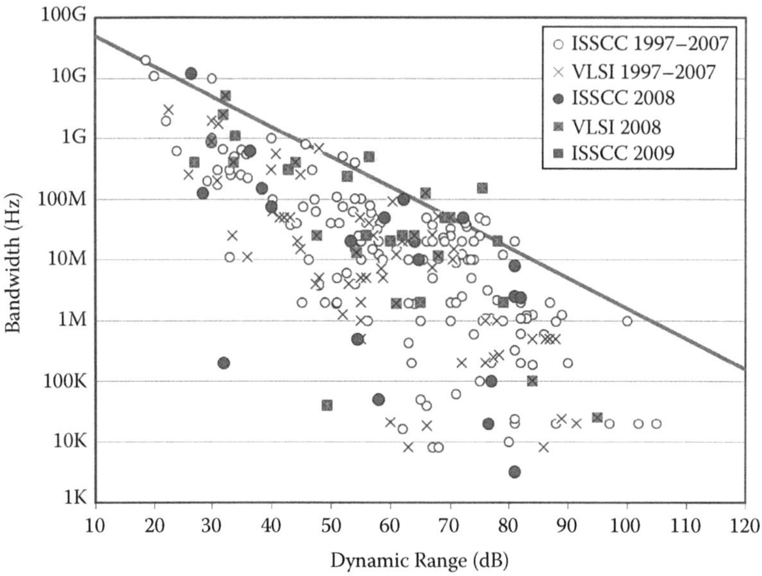

FIGURE 5.3 Dynamic range and bandwidth trends of recently published A/D converters.

Circuits) [18]. The dynamic range and the bandwidth of the A/D converters show an inverse-proportional relationship, and the majority of the recent studies on A/D converters focused on mid-resolution (50–70 dB, i.e., 8–12 bit) and mid-frequency (10–100 MHz) ranges. The requirements for high-resolution (~10 μm minimum feature size), high-frequency (30–150 MHz center frequency of the transducers) ultrasound imaging systems are 50–70 dB dynamic range and 75–400 MHz bandwidth (gray box in the figure). As seen in the figure, a state-of-the-art A/D converter is a fundamental requirement for success of the development of portable high-frequency ultrasound imaging systems.

5.3.3 System Architecture

Novel design architecture is essential to achieve low power consumption, while adapting DBF architecture. DBF architecture consumes considerable power because of the need for a dedicated A/D converter and memory blocks for receive channel. The need for an A/D converter per receive channel in a typical DBF system is a substantial disadvantage because of high power consumption and large system size as compared to an ABF system which delays the received signals, sums them by analog circuitry, and then converts them to a digital signal by an A/D converter.

According to Murmann [19], the power dissipation of the recently published A/D converters in ISSCC and VLSI are about 2×10^{-11} to 2×10^{-8} J at 50 dB dynamic range, as shown in Figure 5.4. For example, assuming the system has 256 receive channels (i.e., it needs 256 A/D converters with DBF architecture), the power

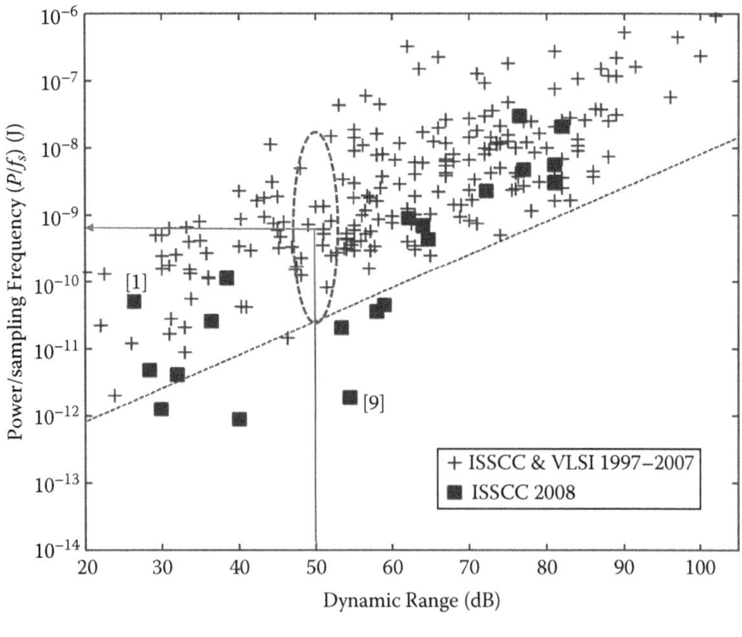

FIGURE 5.4 Power efficiency versus dynamic range in recently published A/D converters.

dissipation of the A/D converter is 5×10^{-10} J (the median value), and the sampling rate is 250 MHz, the system consumes ($32\ \text{W} = 5 \times 10^{-10}\ \text{J} \times 250\ \text{MHz} \times 256$) only for 256 A/D converters. This consumption is rarely practical or even possible considering power consumption limitations in a portable system. For example, the AD9271 chipset has a total of eight receive channels with dedicated A/D converters per each channel and consumes 1.5 W of maximum power. Thus, it needs 48 W of maximum power to build 256 receive channels using the AD9271 chips, which may not be suitable for portable devices.

5.3.3.1 Shared ADC Architecture

To overcome the problem stated previously, the transceiver chip has only one A/D converter shared by the 16 receivers via a 16:1 analog multiplexer (aMUX) as proposed in [9]. Consequently, this configuration creates a DBF system but on the same order of size and power consumption as an ABF system. However, the prototype device operates 16 times slower than a conventional system because the shared ADC architecture performs 16 iterative operations accessing different channels to complete one scan. Another drawback is that the architecture requires extra digital controls.

An evaluation of the effectiveness of the shared ADC architecture, the performance of the shared ADC architecture, and the typical DBF architecture appears as a comparison in Table 5.1. In this comparison, the number of channels in the typical DFB architecture varies from 1 to 16, while the number of channels in the shared ADC architecture remains at 16, and the number of shared channels varies from 4 to 16. The sizes of one receive and transmit channel, an A/D converter, and the 3 Kb SRAM are assumed to be 0.175, 0.9, and 2.16 mm^2, respectively. These sizes are estimates based on the actual layout sizes of each component in the transceiver chip. The size of digital control circuitry, needed only for the shared ADC architecture, is expected to be 0.2 mm^2. In addition, the assumed power consumption of one receive and transmit channel, an A/D converter, 3 Kb SRAM, and the digital controls are 2, 100, 130, and 8 mW, respectively. These data were also estimated from SPICE simulation results of each component with post-layout parameters. The time for 1-scanning is calculated based on the operational sequence and time for

TABLE 5.1
Performance Comparison among Shared ADC and Typical DBF Architectures

	Typical DBF Architecture			Shared ADC Architecture		
	Number of Channels			Number of Shared Channels[a]		
	1	**8**	**16**	**4**	**8**	**16**
Numbers of required ADC and SRAM	1	8	16	4	2	1
Chip size (mm^2)	3.24	25.9	51.8	15.2	9.1	6.1
Power consumption (mW)	240	1864	3720	960	500	270
Time for 1-scanning (μs)	50	50	50	200	400	800

[a] Total number of channels: 16.

one complete scanning of the Penn State ultrasound imaging system described in Section 5.4.

Table 5.1 also indicates the trade-off relationship among operational speed for 1-scanning, chip size, and power consumption. Thus, to determine an optimal number of shared channels, the maximum time for 1-complete scanning allowed for real-time imaging is a consideration. Having established the maximum time, the total number of channels can be determined considering the chip size and power consumption specifications. For example, if the maximum allowable time for 1-scanning is 800 μs, the 16 channels can be shared. Then, if the chip size is 25 mm^2 and power consumption is 1 W, the optimal number of total channels will be 64 (16 channels of each are shared).

5.4 PENN STATE PORTABLE HIGH-FREQUENCY ULTRASOUND IMAGING SYSTEM

5.4.1 Configuration of the Penn State Ultrasound Imaging System

Conventional front-end electronics consist of discrete chipsets for transmitters, preamplifiers, TGCs, A/D converters, and memory devices, all mounted on several PCBs (printed circuit boards). Therefore, the systems are not only large and expensive but they also have difficulty with high-speed operation. The Penn State ultrasound imaging system integrates the complete ultrasound front-end electronics onto a single IC chip with closed-coupled thin-film ultrasound transducers, and then constructs high-resolution ultrasound images. The system requires (1) a multichannel analog signal processing system including high-speed A/D converters and a transmit beamformer integrated on a single transceiver chip, and (2) auxiliary digital controls on an FPGA (field programmable gate array) chip with several discrete chipsets such as an RS-232 chip, a D/A converter (DAC), and a 250 MHz crystal oscillator. These specifications enable creation of an ultra-compact, low-cost, high-speed, and high-resolution ultrasound imaging system.

The FPGA chip has been programmed to control the ultrasound transceiver chip, and helps the transceiver chip to communicate with the imaging host via an RS-232 chip. The main control interfaces with other circuitry such as mode set, memory, and the transceiver chip according to commands received from the user. The clock buffer receives a 250 MHz clock signal from an external clock oscillator and distributes it to other circuit blocks and to the transceiver chip. The mode set consists of 1 bit serial pipeline registers that store data preset by the user, for example, channel and the preamplifier gain selection information. The 48 Kb internal memory's assignment is to store image information from the transceiver chip. The stored data, transferred to the host computer through the serial port in the FPGA chip and the RS-232 chip, allows subsequent image creation. The counter's design permits generation of digital codes that increase as an exponential function of time. The digital codes produce a pseudo-exponential analog signal for the VGA in the transceiver chip.

Figure 5.5 shows a block diagram of the transceiver chip. The receiver consists of a preamplifier and a TGC that compensates for signal attenuation as a function of depth. The TGC consists of an on-chip VGA and an external 10 bit 50 MHz

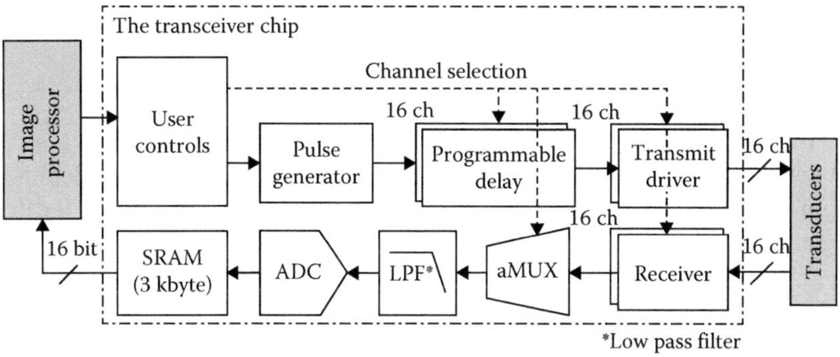

FIGURE 5.5 Simplified block diagram of the transceiver chip.

D/A converter (AD9760, Analog Devices, Wilmington, MA). A time-varying control signal, applied to the VGA gain control input, ensures the signal strength at the VGA output is constant over time (i.e., depth). An 8 bit A/D converter digitizes the compensated signals. The A/D converter output connects to a 3 Kb on-chip SRAM, which is large enough to store all the scanned image data for a specified depth range. In this work, the transceiver chip has 16 transmit and receive channels. The number of channels can be increased. The transceiver chip has only one A/D converter and SRAM to reduce chip area and power consumption, but the system needs an analog multiplexer (aMUX) and auxiliary digital controls for channel selection. A 16:1 analog multiplexer allows these two components to share 16 receive channels. The next subsection discusses the architectural advantage of the transceiver chip.

The transmit signal generator produces and sends a 50 MHz pulse to the thin-film ultrasound transducers through programmable delay chains to enable electronic beam focusing in the transmit mode. In a DBF system, focusing occurs by introducing delays to the transmit pulse on the elements so that emitted ultrasonic beams can be made constructively at the target of interest. Therefore, excitation pulses should be delivered to the transducer elements in an order that allows convergence of a composite wave front at a point. The variable delay chains in the figure determine the excitation order of the transducers.

5.4.2 Receiver

5.4.2.1 Required Specifications

The most important design specification of the system is the bandwidth of the receiver. The required bandwidth of the receiver is determined by the center frequency and bandwidth of the transducer. In this study, the target frequency of the transducers is 50 MHz with 100% bandwidth; thus, the input frequency range is 25–75 MHz [16]. Therefore, the receiver circuitry must be capable of a flat frequency response over the bandwidth of the transducer elements up to 75 MHz with a maximum gain of 20 dB.

In addition, the ratio of the A/D converter aperture and the maximum preamplifier input amplitude determines the gain of the preamplifier according to

$$Gain_{preamp} = 20 \cdot \log_{10}\left(\frac{Max\ ADC\ input}{Max\ Preamp\ input}\right) \pm (Design\ margin) \tag{5.4}$$

In this design, the maximum input of the preamplifier is set to 0.3 V_{P_P}, and the A/D converter aperture is 1.5 V_{P_P}. Thus, the preamplifier gain is 14 dB ± (design margin). Since the thin-film transducers are currently under development, the design margin is set to ± 6 dB. Therefore, the gain of the preamplifier can be changed over a range from 8 to 20 dB at the discretion of the user.

The dynamic range of the preamplifier is another important factor in the receive circuitry. The dynamic range of the receiver determines the minimum and the maximum signal amplitudes that the system can process. Therefore, the attenuation rate and depth range of the target medium can determine the required dynamic range. Assuming the attenuation rate in soft tissue is 0.5 dB/MHz/cm [20], the total attenuation is 45 dB at 50 MHz for a penetration depth of 9 mm (i.e., the total signal path of 18 mm considering signal reflection). Adding a minimum display resolution of 30 dB, image saturation allowance of 6 dB, and noise threshold of 6 dB [21] provides a dynamic range of 87 dB [22]. Therefore, the SNR (signal-to-noise ratio) of the A/D converter needs to be greater than 87 dB, which corresponds to 15 bit resolution, according to the relationship [21]

$$SNR_{ideal} = 6.02N + 1.76(dB) \tag{5.5}$$

where N is the bit resolution of an A/D converter.

However, this dynamic range is too great for current high-speed A/D converters. The use of a VGA reduces the dynamic range requirement. Since the main purpose of the VGA is to compensate signal attenuation as a function of the depth of targets, the maximum gain of the VGA is bounded by the total signal attenuation, that is, 45 dB. The optimal gain range of the VGA is selectable according to the dynamic range of the A/D converter. For example, if the SNR of the A/D converter is 42 dB, 45 dB of variable gain range is the requirement. In this design, the target SNR of the A/D converter is 48 dB (i.e., 8 bit); thus, the required gain range of the VGA is 37 dB. Figure 5.6 illustrates the gain and dynamic range requirements.

5.4.2.2 Circuit Design Details

The receive circuitry consists of two on-chip components (the preamp and the VGA) and several off-chip components. The counter included in the FPGA chip generates time-varying digital codes that convert to the pseudo-exponential analog control signals through an external D/A converter. The VGA can produce a time-varying gain on a linear decibel scale with pseudo-exponential control signals.

Figure 5.7 shows the simplified circuit schematic of the preamplifier. The analog signals from the transducers connect to IN+ and the common ground of the transducer arrays connects to IN–. The resistance ratio of the transistors M1 and M2 and the resistors R1 and R2 determine the gain. Expression of the voltage gain of the amplifier is

$$A_V = -g_{m1,2} \cdot (r_{O1,2} \| r_{O3,4} \| R_{1,2}) \tag{5.6}$$

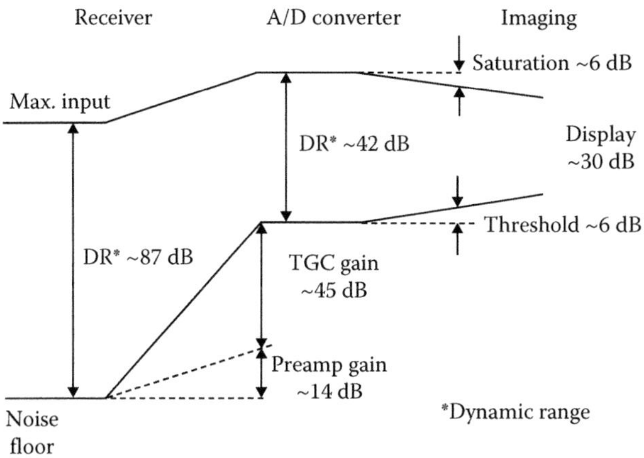

FIGURE 5.6 Transceiver chip gain and dynamic range requirements.

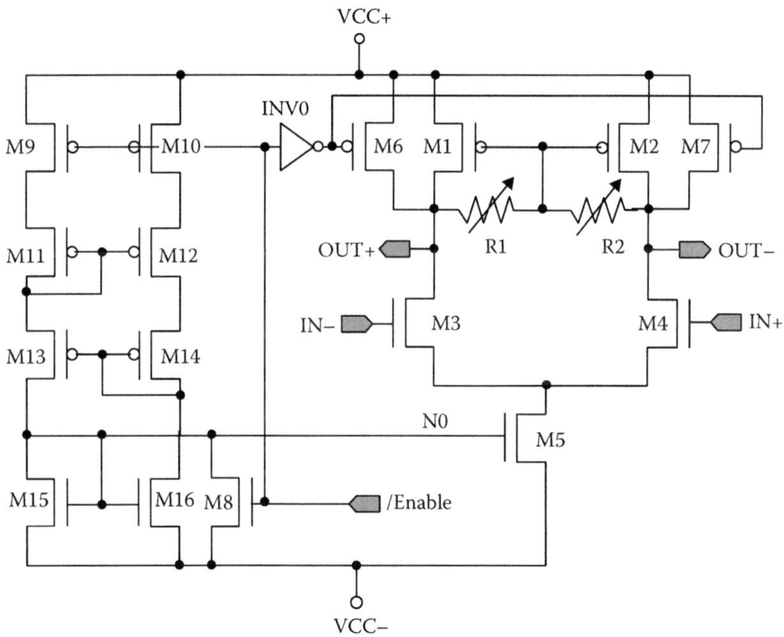

FIGURE 5.7 Preamplifier core circuit schematic.

where

- $g_{m1,2}$ is the transconductance of M1 and M2
- $r_{O1,2}$ is the output resistances of the transistors M1 and M2
- $r_{O3,4}$ is the output resistances of transistors M3 and M4
- R1 and R2 in the design vary the resistance value from 4 to 20 KΩ so that the user can preset the gain

The combination of transistors M6–M10 and inverter INV0 form the enable/disable switch. This internal switch eliminates external T/R switches (required in typical ultrasound transceivers) in the analog signal path. When "/Enable" is HIGH, transistor M8 turns OFF so that the voltage of the node N_0 goes to ground, and transistors M6 and M7 turn ON so that OUT+ and OUT– are tied to VCC+ regardless of the amplifier's inputs. The speed of the switch is fast enough for the amplifier to be stable before signal acquisition starts. Transistors M9–M16 generate bias voltages, independent of the power supply voltages, for the amplifier.

Since an ultrasound wave attenuates its power traveling in tissue on a decibel scale, the gain of the VGA also needs to have the capability to be changed linearly in dB [20]. Therefore, the gain of the VGA must be linear-in-dB over the linear control voltage range. To achieve this relationship, the proposed design adapts a Gilbert-type four-quadrant multiplier, whose output is equal to the product of the two inputs [23], and the generated pseudo-exponential control voltages use external circuitry with an FPGA chip and a D/A converter. Figure 5.8 depicts the folded Gilbert cell, in which the bottom differential pair of the original Gilbert cell folds without degrading performance in order to reduce the number of cascode transistors. Derivation of the analytic relationship between input and output is [24]

$$\begin{aligned} Vo &= (g_{m3,4} - g_{m5,6}) \cdot R_D \cdot (V_{\text{in+}} - V_{\text{in-}}) \\ &= \sqrt{\frac{k_n (W/L)}{2I_{SS}}} \cdot g_{m1,2} (V_{\text{cp}} - V_{\text{cn}})(V_{\text{in+}} - V_{\text{in-}}) \end{aligned} \tag{5.7}$$

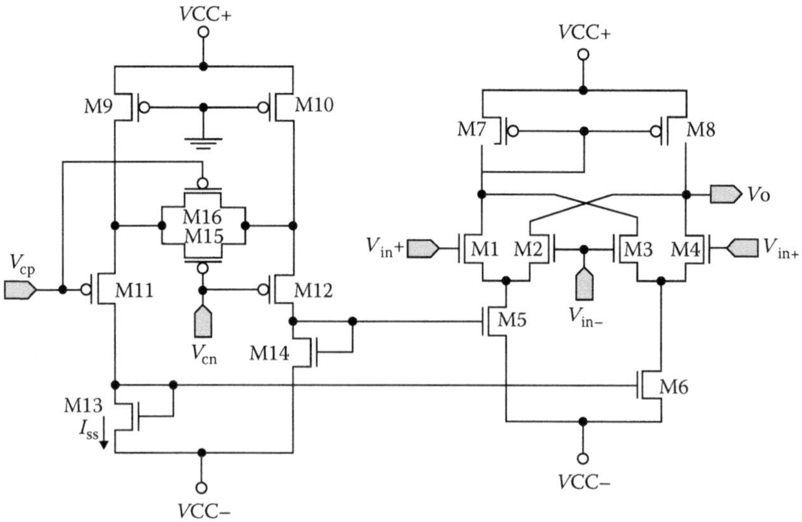

FIGURE 5.8 Folded Gilbert cell–based VGA circuit schematic.

where

$g_{m1,2}$, $g_{m3,4}$, and $g_{m5,6}$ are the transconductances of transistors M1 and M2, M3 and M4, and M5 and M6, respectively

$k_N = \mu_N \cdot C_{ox}$ (μ_N is the electron mobility and C_{ox} is the gate capacitance of the NMOS transistor)

W is the channel width of transistors M1–M4

L is the channel length of transistors M1–M4

Transistors M9–M16 constitute a linear voltage converter.

Figure 5.9 presents the measured output of the receive circuitry including the preamplifier and the VGA. The preamplifier gain is set to 14 dB and the linear gain control range of the VGA is 23 dB with control voltage of 0.1–1.0 V, which is generated using the FPGA chip (Spartan III, Xilinx, Inc.) and a 10 bit D/A converter (AD 9760, Analog Devices, Inc.). The results demonstrate the function of the receiver: the amplitude of the second and the third peaks is similar to that of the first peak due to the increasing gain over the time.

5.4.3 A/D Converter

The sampling rate of the A/D converter can be determined by the Nyquist sampling theorem [25], which states that reconstruction of a continuous-time signal from its samples is possible if the sampling frequency is greater than twice the signal bandwidth. If the center frequency of the target transducer is 50 MHz with 100% bandwidth, the bandwidth of the reflected signals will be 25–75 MHz. Given the 20 MHz design margin of the anti-aliasing filter located between the VGA and the A/D converter, the signal bandwidth will be 5–95 MHz. Therefore, the required

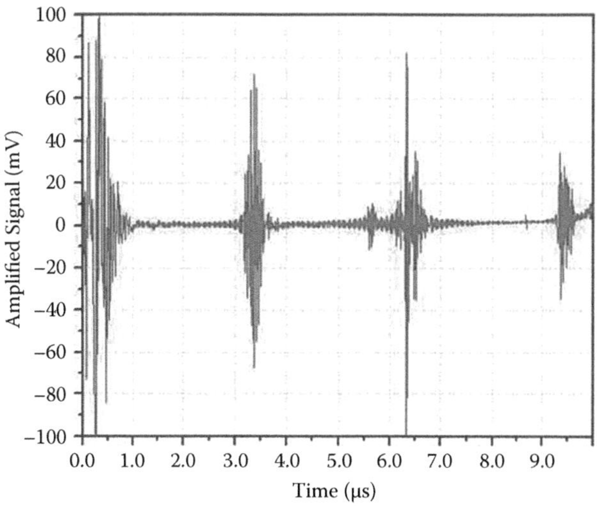

FIGURE 5.9 Amplified signals by the receiver with the VGA functioning. These results were obtained with the test board shown in Figure 5.19.

minimum sampling rate of the A/D converter is 190 MHz according to the Nyquist theorem.

A further important determination is the effective bit resolution. This consideration depends on the characteristics of the medium. In this design, the target medium is tissue in human organs, which requires at least a 50 dB image resolution [21]. Therefore, the required effective bit resolution of the A/D converter is set to 50 dB, that is, an 8 bit resolution.

5.4.3.1 TIQ-Based A/D Converter

The design of a 190 MS/s A/D converter is a challenge in 0.35 μm CMOS technology. To achieve the A/D converter requirements, a TIQ (threshold inverter quantization) A/D converter (TIQ ADC), known for its fast conversion speed [26], has been designed. Although a flash-type A/D converter has several disadvantages in terms of higher power consumption, occupying a larger area than other types of A/D converters, the shared A/D converter architecture described in Section 5.3 overcomes the drawbacks of the flash A/D converter. Since this architecture, reportedly, has the operation speed, gain, and DC offset variations of up to 18% due to process and temperature variations [26], a sampling rate of 250 MHz rather than the required sampling rate of 190 MHz is the target for the proposed design.

A TIQ comparator is one of the most important circuits in a flash A/D converter. It converts an analog input voltage into a digital logic output "1" or "0," depending on the reference voltage of the comparator. In a traditional flash A/D converter, a differential comparator, which needs a resistor-ladder circuit as an external voltage reference, is commonly used. On the other hand, the TIQ comparator, which consists of two cascaded CMOS inverters, does not need a resistor-ladder circuit because it uses the built-in voltage reference of the CMOS inverters [27].

As an example of TIQ ADC operation, Figure 5.10a shows the schematic of a 2 bit TIQ ADC comprising 3 TIQ comparators, 3 gain boosters, and 1 encoder (notably, an n bit TIQ ADC consists of $2^n - 1$ comparators and gain boosters and an n bit encoder). The TIQ comparator consists of two cascaded inverters: the first inverter sets the analog signal quantization according to its logic threshold, and the second inverter increases the gain of the comparator. If the analog input is higher than the logic threshold, the digital output is logic "1"; otherwise, the digital output is logic "0."

A particular output voltage (V_{out}) that is the same as input voltage (V_{in}), that is, $V_{in} = V_{out}$, determines the logic threshold of the TIQ comparator. And the logic threshold changes depending on the width ratios of the PMOS and NMOS. If P1 is the largest PMOS and P5 is the smallest PMOS, and if N1 is the smallest NMOS and N5 is the largest PMOS, as shown in Figure 5.10a, the top comparator output corresponds to C_3; the middle comparator corresponds to C_2; and the bottom comparator output corresponds to C_1 as in Figure 5.10b. Clearly, the three different ratios of the PMOS and NMOS widths result in three different logic thresholds: the logic threshold value of the top comparator is the largest and the logic threshold of the bottom comparator is the smallest.

With fixed lengths for the PMOS and NMOS transistors, increasing or decreasing the width of the PMOS or NMOS, respectively, produces the desired values for the logic thresholds. Since the TIQ comparator is used in a flash A/D converter, a $2^n - 1$ set of TIQ comparators is necessary to design an n bit flash A/D converter.

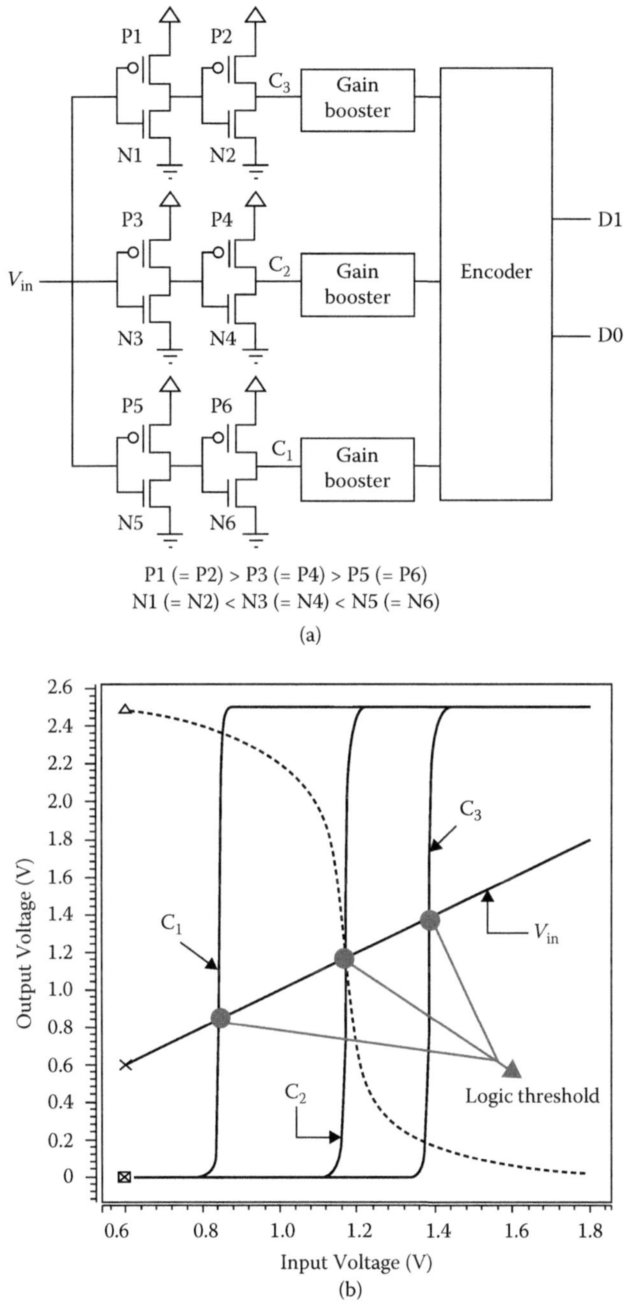

FIGURE 5.10 TIQ comparator design: (a) example of 2 bit TIQ A/D converter, (b) VTC of a TIQ comparator.

Therefore, finding the exact $2^n - 1$ different logic thresholds as the reference voltages of the TIQ comparator in an input voltage range is necessary. For example, all 63 TIQ comparators for a 6 bit flash A/D converter have transistors of different sizes, so all the comparators have different logic threshold values.

5.4.3.2 Design Automation for the TIQ Comparator

The simple architecture of TIQ ADC is an advantage; however, for a TIQ ADC, the TIQ comparators' design must be precisely sized to be different from one another. Achieving the required dynamic range makes designing this feature a somewhat difficult task. Mitigating the difficulty is use of a CAD (computer aided design) tool, which automates TIQ comparator design and implementation. The systematic size variation (SSV) technique is the proposed method for easing, comparatively, the choice of needed logic thresholds from the many possible comparators [27]. The SSV technique chooses V_m from a reduced range of 3-D plots. The diagonal line drawn in the 3-D plots is the optimal line, which maintains a systematic increasing and/or decreasing order of transistor sizes. Keeping the transistor size in increasing and/or decreasing order significantly improves the linearity of the A/D converter in relationship to CMOS process variation. This method also significantly reduces the number of simulations needed for transistor size selection. The simulation is needed only along the diagonal-line region rather than on the full 3-D surface.

Using the SSV could save this design time. However, it is still time-consuming due to simulating all possible combinations of the PMOS and NMOS. For example, according to [28], about 4 h were necessary to find 6 bit TIQ comparators using the SSV technique, and 5 Sun-Blade 2000 machines performed 28,000 simulations to find 63 TIQ comparators. Notably, the total design time increases exponentially if the bit resolution of a TIQ ADC increases.

An improved TIQ comparator design methodology has been proposed in [28]. The proposed method introduces an analytical TIQ model to overcome the drawbacks of the SSV technique. The analytical model has advantages over the SSV technique in terms of simulation time as well as accuracy.

Since the logic threshold (V_m) is a voltage in which the output voltage is equal to the input voltage ($V_{out} = V_{in} = V_m$), mathematical expression of V_m can be derived from drain current equations for both PMOS and NMOS devices. For simplicity, only a TIQ model using a Level 1 SPICE model has been derived here. More sophisticated models, such as BSIM3 (Berkeley Short-channel IGFET Model) or BSIM4 [29], may improve the model's accuracy. Also, the assumption is that the channel lengths of PMOS and NMOS devices are long enough; that is, velocity saturation does not occur. The drain currents of NMOS and PMOS, $I_{DS,NMOS}$, $I_{DS,PMOS}$, respectively, can be denoted

$$I_{DS,NMOS} = \frac{k_N}{2}\left(\frac{W_N}{L_N}\right)(V_m - V_{THN})^2(1+\lambda_N V_{DS}) \tag{5.8}$$

$$I_{DS,PMOS} = \frac{k_P}{2}\left(\frac{W_P}{L_P}\right)(V_{DD} - V_m - |V_{THP}|)^2(1+\lambda_P V_{DS}) \tag{5.9}$$

where

$k_N = \mu_N \cdot C_{OXN}$ (μ_N is the electron mobility and C_{OXN} is the gate capacitance of NMOS)

$k_P = \mu_P \cdot C_{OXP}$ (μ_P is the hole mobility and C_{OXP} is the gate capacitance of PMOS)

When the channel lengths of both transistors are the same, the logic threshold, V_m, yields

$$V_m = \frac{V_{THN} + (V_{DD} - |V_{THP}|) \cdot \Lambda \cdot \sqrt{k_P W_P / k_N W_N}}{1 + \sqrt{k_P W_P / k_N W_N}} \tag{5.10}$$

where $\Lambda = \sqrt{2 + \lambda_P V_{DD} / 2 + \lambda_N V_{DD}}$.

From Equation (5.10), the dependency of V_m on the width ratio of the PMOS and NMOS (W_P/W_N) can be derived. Figure 5.11 shows the comparison of V_m dependencies on the width ratios in analytical models and the SSV technique. A standard 0.35 μm CMOS technology is used for this graph, and the SSV technique generates a set of 63 TIQ comparators for a 6 bit TIQ ADC. The V_m curve from the BSIM3 model shows excellent accuracy with an average mismatch rate of less than 1%. The maximum error is about 5%, and the average error is less than 1%. Therefore, a set of width ratios, according to ideal V_m values, can be found using the TIQ model rather than the SSV technique.

As an alternate form of Equation (5.10), a set of widths can be expressed as a function of V_m. This alternate set is

$$\left(\frac{W_P}{W_N}\right) = \frac{k_N (V_m - V_{THN})^2 (2 + \lambda_N V_{DD})}{k_P (V_{DD} - V_m - |V_{THP}|)^2 (2 + \lambda_P V_{DD})} \tag{5.11}$$

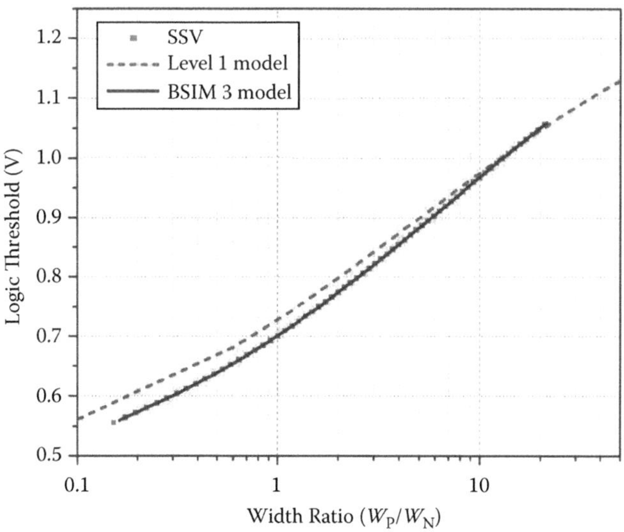

FIGURE 5.11 Accuracy comparison of various TIQ comparator models.

Equation (5.11) provides the width ratio for each ideal V_m. The width ratios of the TIQ comparators can be expressed as

$$\frac{W_P(i)}{W_N(i)} = R(i), \quad (i = 1\text{-}2^n - 1) \tag{5.12}$$

where

$W_P(i)$ is the i_{th} PMOS width
$W_N(i)$ is the i_{th} NMOS width
$R(i)$ is the i_{th} width ratio for the n bit TIQ comparator set

However, determining the widths of NMOS and PMOS devices cannot occur using only Equation (5.12) without another relationship between W_P and W_N. The relationship arises from the projection of the line on the x–y plane, as illustrated in Figure 5.12. The line expression, in a general form, is

$$a \cdot W_P + b \cdot W_N = c \tag{5.13}$$

where a, b, and c are constants. In the case of process variation, shifting the NMOS and PMOS at the same ratio is desirable. Thus, the a and b can be set to 1. Therefore, (5.13) can be denoted as

$$W_P(i) + W_N(i) = k \tag{5.14}$$

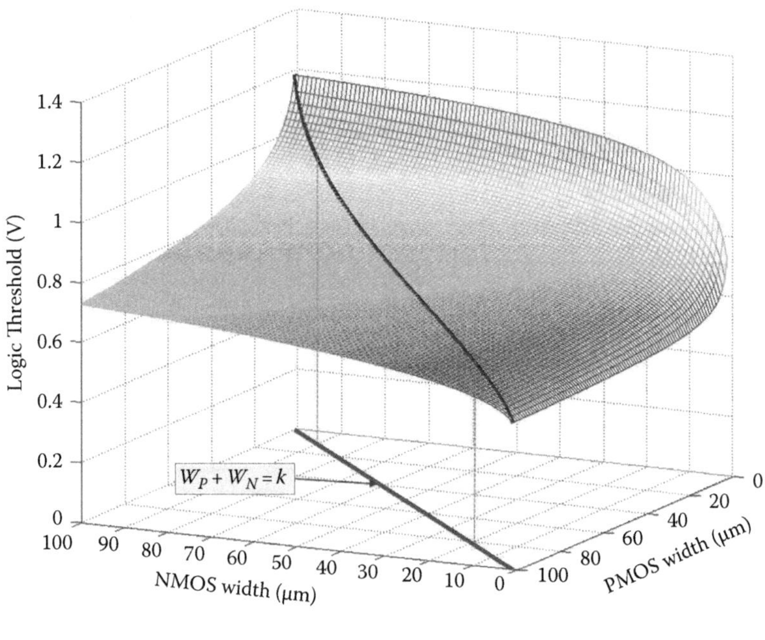

FIGURE 5.12 3-D plot of V_m and the width size relationship of the NMOS and the PMOS of the TIQ comparator analytical model.

From Equations (5.12) and (5.14), $W_P(i)$ and $W_N(i)$ can be derived as

$$W_P(i) = \frac{k \cdot R(i)}{1 + R(i)} \tag{5.15}$$

and

$$W_N(i) = \frac{k}{1 + R(i)} \tag{5.16}$$

The optimal transistor length parameters are derived from considering the relationship between transistor length and data conversion speed. In general, a longer transistor length in a TIQ comparator is desirable for achieving higher gain, that is, higher sensitivity, less noise, and less process variation sensitivity. However, a longer transistor yields a slower data comparison speed in the TIQ comparator. If the conversion target speed is 1 GSPS, a maximum transistor length of about 1 μm is allowed in a 0.18 μm standard CMOS technology [28]. Consequently, the optimal value of the transistor length in a TIQ comparator can be set to 1 μm for a 1-GSPS TIQ ADC.

5.4.4 SRAM

5.4.4.1 Required Specifications

The SRAM included in the design reduces the data transfer rates from the A/D converter to the imaging host processor. Since the sampling rate of the A/D converter is 250 MS/s and the bit resolution is 8 bits, the digitized image data transfers to the host at the data bandwidth of 2 GBPS. However, such high-speed data transfer is not only difficult to be achieved using less expensive circuit boards but it also generates substantial digital noise (jitters) that negatively affects the analog signal integrity of the receiver. On-chip memory devices overcome these problems. Therefore, an SRAM that can write data with a data bandwidth of 2 GBPS and that can read data with a lower data transfer rate of 250 MBPS became elements of the design for the CMOS transceiver chip.

Another key specification of the on-chip memory is capacity. The calculation of the memory capacity uses the relationship

$$Capacity = \frac{t_{Travel}}{t_{sample}} = \frac{D / c}{t_{sample}} \tag{5.17}$$

where

t_{Travel} is the total (i.e., two way) travel time of the ultrasound wave in the medium
t_{sample} is the sampling interval of the A/D converter
D is the total distance that the ultrasound wave travels in the medium
c is the speed of the ultrasound wave in the medium

Estimates indicate that a 3-Kb buffer length is necessary for $t_{\text{sample}} = 4$ ns, $D = 18$ mm, and $c = 1500$ m/s.

5.4.4.2 SRAM Design Details

Figure 5.13 shows the functional block diagram of a 3 Kb SRAM. This SRAM operates in two modes: data write mode and data read mode with auto precharge. Once the data write or data read operation begins, the operation continues until the all 3 Kb cells are written to or read by the address counter, which automatically, incrementally sweeps all 3000 addresses.

The SRAM design adopts asymmetric operating speed between data write and data read. As described earlier, the data write speed is faster than 125 MHz; however, a 125 MHz data readout speed could be a disaster in some inexpensive applications. Thus, this design uses two different speed clocks for data write and data read. First, a 250 MHz clock is used for data conversion and storing. Next, a 50 MHz clock is used for the system I/O. Thus, the data readout uses the 50 MHz clock. The main I/O clock offers an inexpensive and easy way of transferring data.

The asymmetric operating speed between data write and data read occurs by a 2:1 multiplexer. During write operations, the SRAM shares the A/D converter clock, and the SRAM uses the main I/O clock during the readout operation. Figure 5.14 presents the SPICE simulation results of the SRAM clock transition. Until 700 ns, the SRAM writes the data in the memory cells in the two subbanks with a 250 MHz clock speed as shown in Figure 5.14b and c. Clearly, the subbanks operate one after the other as mentioned earlier. At 700 ns, the read command comes in, and the clock changes from 250 to 50 MHz. Thus, the read operation performs with the 50 MHz clock.

Figure 5.15 presents the measured outputs of the SRAM, which transferred at a rate of 400 MBPS as described earlier. In this figure, only 6 bit outputs are presented because the A/D converter shows linear characteristics with 6 bits. An 85 kHz of sawtooth wave was generated by a function generator and fed to the A/D converter. The analog signal was sampled at a speed of 250 MS/s, then converted to digital signals. The SRAM stored the digital data at the same speed as the A/D converter's sampling rate. The test results prove the functionality of the SRAM and the A/D converter.

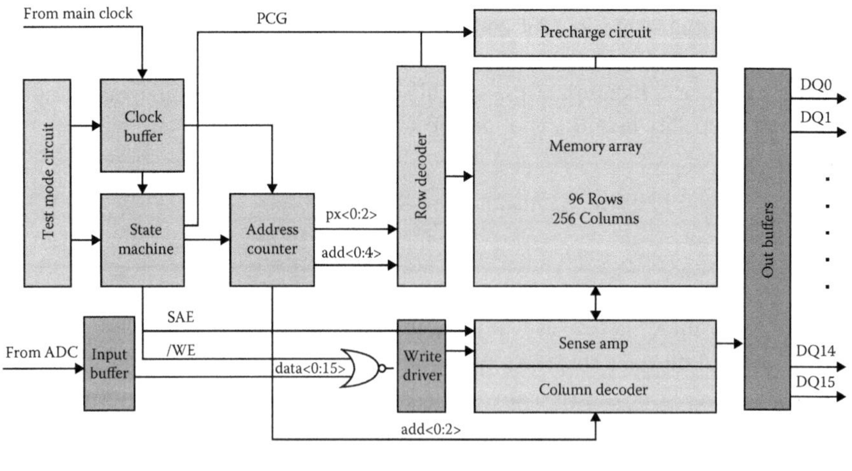

FIGURE 5.13 Functional block diagram of the 3 Kb SRAM.

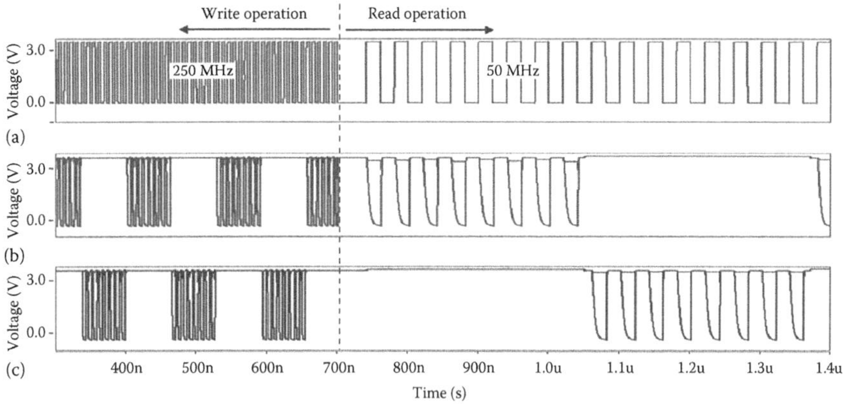

FIGURE 5.14 Simulation results of the SRAM clock modulation: (a) clock transition, (b) memory cell data in Bank 0, (c) memory cell data in Bank 1.

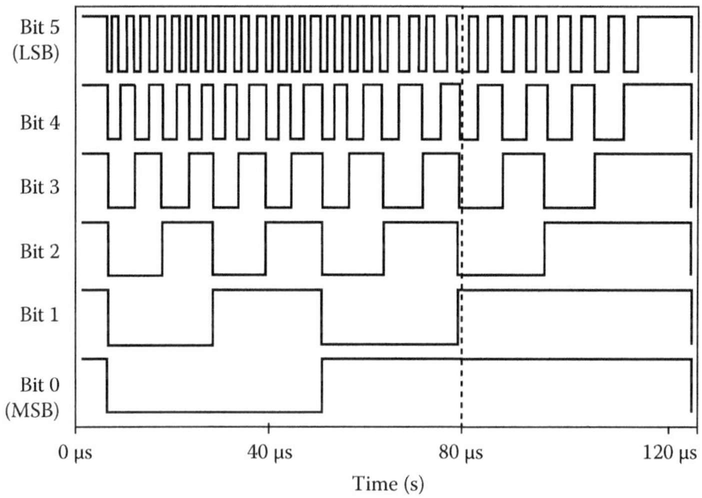

FIGURE 5.15 Measured outputs of the SRAM with the transfer rate of 400 MBPS.

5.4.5 Transmitter

The major function of the transmitter is to excite the transducer elements and to focus and/or steer the ultrasound beam. Focusing and steering the ultrasonic beam requires time delays to compensate for the acoustic signal path length differences from the transducer array to the target of interest. The expression for the focused signal $f(t)$ is

$$f(t) = \sum_{n=-N/2}^{n=N/2} X_n(t - \tau_n) \tag{5.18}$$

where

N is the total number of transducer elements

X_n is the received reflected signal

τ_n is channel delay time for the nth transducer element [15]

The delay time, τ_n, derives from Figure 5.16. Assuming a signal, transmitted with the steering angle θ by exciting a transducer located at 0, a reflected signal propagates back from the focal point to the transducer array. When the distance from the focal point to the transducer center is R, the distance from the focal point to the nth transducer has the expression: $L + R$, as shown in Figure 5.16. By denoting the space between adjacent channels, d, expression of the channel delays is

$$\tau_n = \tau_n(R) = \frac{R}{c}\left[\sqrt{1+\left(\frac{nd}{R}\right)^2 + 2\left(\frac{nd}{R}\right)\sin\theta} - 1\right] \quad (5.19)$$

where c is the average propagation speed of ultrasound in the medium [30].

The design of the programmable delays provides different delay times for each of the elements in a 16 × 1 array configuration. Implementing such a fine delay step in a CMOS technology is challenging in beamformer design. The most recently designed digital clock delay schemes use PLLs (phase locked loops) [15,30]. However, a 20 ps delay step would need at least a 10-GHz clock using these methods. This is not feasible in a 0.35 μm standard CMOS technology. Therefore, this work adopts an analog delay chain method. Figure 5.17 is a block diagram of the proposed delay chain. One of five delay buffers can be selected for coarse delay time setting with a 100-ps step. Then four different loading options can be added for the 20 ps fine delay step. Every channel on the chip has the channel delay setting circuit; therefore, a host

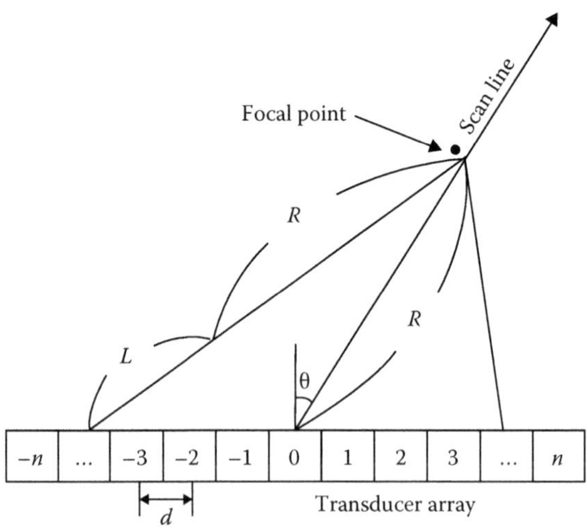

FIGURE 5.16 Dynamic focusing and steering delay.

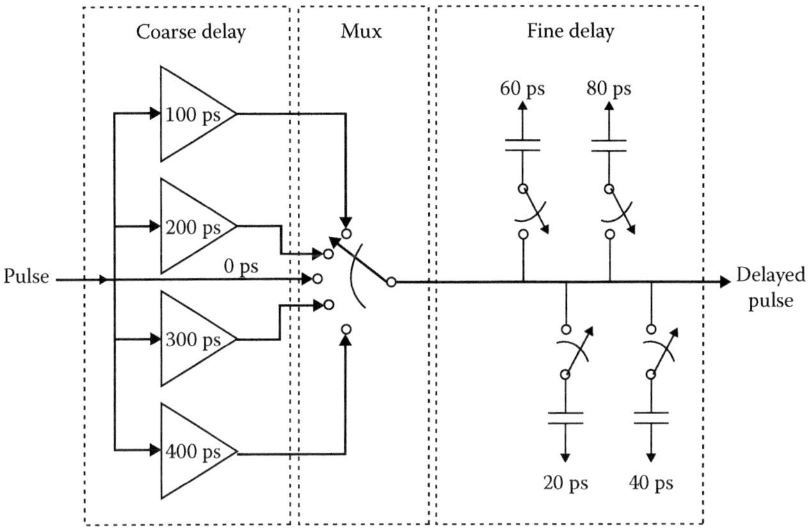

FIGURE 5.17 Circuit schematic of programmable delays for beam focusing.

computer can control delays between pulses by transmit beam focusing. Although required channel delays are 20–160 ps, the channel delays are programmable from 20 to 480 ps in order to compensate for the initial channel delay mismatch.

Figure 5.18 illustrates the transmit pulses generated by the transceiver chip. The transmit pulses can be delayed from 20 to 500 ps as described in the previous section. The delays by the programmable delay chain in the chip are measured with a high-precision digital oscilloscope (Agilent Infiniium 8000). Notably, the signals shown in the figure are calibrated to compensate for the initial channel delays due to signal line mismatches on the printed circuit board. The frequency of the pulses can be varied from 1 to 100 MHz, where 5 MHz pulses are shown in the figure.

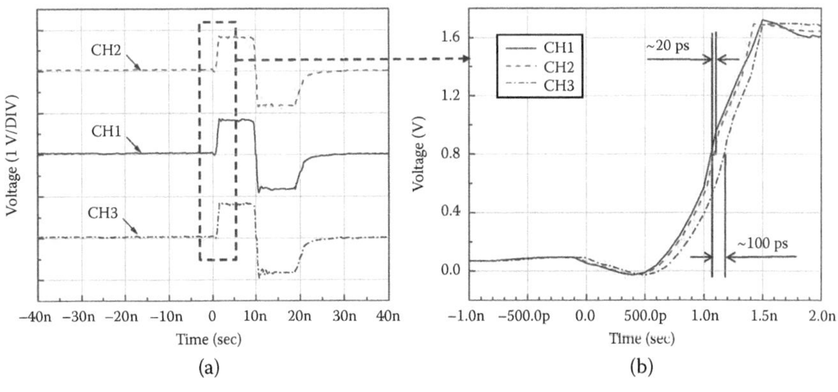

FIGURE 5.18 Measured delay of transmit channels: (a) transmit pulses with various channel delays (50 MHz), (b) magnified view of the box in blank on (a).

5.4.6 Experimental Results

5.4.6.1 Prototype Experimental Board

The transceiver chip was fabricated using a TSMC 0.35 μm, double-poly, four-metal process through MOSIS. The die size was 10 mm^2. Figure 5.19 shows the mounting of the transceiver chip and the thin-film transducers on test board (a), and a microphotograph of the first-generation transceiver chip (b). The average power consumption in the receive mode, consisting of 16 receiver channels, A/D converter, and SRAM, operating simultaneously, is approximately 270 mW with a 3.3 V power supply. The shared A/D converter and SRAM architecture, which reduced the number of A/D converters and SRAMs from 16 to 1, resulted in smaller chip area and lower power consumption. This size and power consumption are reasonable for a portable ultrasound imaging system using the transceiver chip; they can be decreased further if a state-of-the-art process technology, for example, a 90 nm or 0.13 μm CMOS process technology, is used. Table 5.2 summarizes the specifications for the transceiver chip.

5.4.6.2 Thin-Film Ultrasound Transducer Array

T-bar-shaped ultrasound PZT ($PbZr_{0.52}Ti_{0.48}O_3$) transducer arrays have been developed and documented in [16]. PZT layers can be thin, and allow reduction of the required voltages for exciting the transducer. Therefore, directly driving the transducers with low-voltage CMOS signals is possible. The thin-film transducers' fabrication employed a Sol–gel and multilayer dry-etching process. Ti/Pt bottom electrodes were deposited on a silicon wafer on which a 300 nm thermal silicon-dioxide film was preformed. The total of 0.5–0.6 μm PZT films was deposited using the Sol–gel process over the bottom electrode; then, Pt top electrodes were formed. Finally, the T-bar shape transducer array structure was patterned by dry-etching. Figure 5.20 shows an SEM (scanning electron microscopy) image of the transducer array (a) and its frequency spectrum (b). The dimensions of a T-bar structure are 30 μm in width and 300 μm in length. Details of the thin-film transducers have reference in [16]. The target, center frequency of the thin-film transducer is 30–70 MHz, and that of the particular transducer array in these experiments is 35 MHz, with a

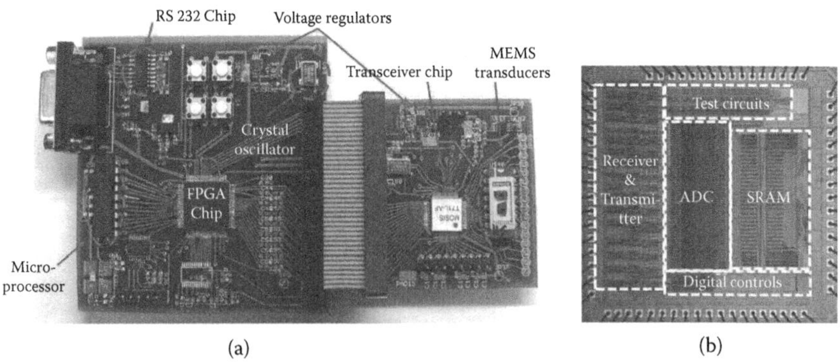

FIGURE 5.19 (a) Test board for the transceiver chip with the thin film transducer array, (b) microphotograph of the CMOS transceiver chip.

TABLE 5.2
CMOS Transceiver Chip Specifications Summary

Preamp	Gain (dB)	5–20
	Bandwidth (MHz)	>75
	Dynamic range (dB)	90
	Noise figure (dB)	10
VGA	Gain range (dB)	46
	Bandwidth (MHz)	250
	Noise figure (dB)	6–12
ADC	Resolution (bit)	6
	Conversion speed (MHz)	250
Memory	Capacity (byte)	3K
	Data bandwidth (MBPS)	250
Transmitter	Pulse frequency (MHz)	1–100
	Delay step (ps)	20
Total chip	Noise figure (dB)	9.7–14.5
	Power consumption	270 mW
	Process technology	TSMC 0.35 μm
	Chip size	10 mm^2

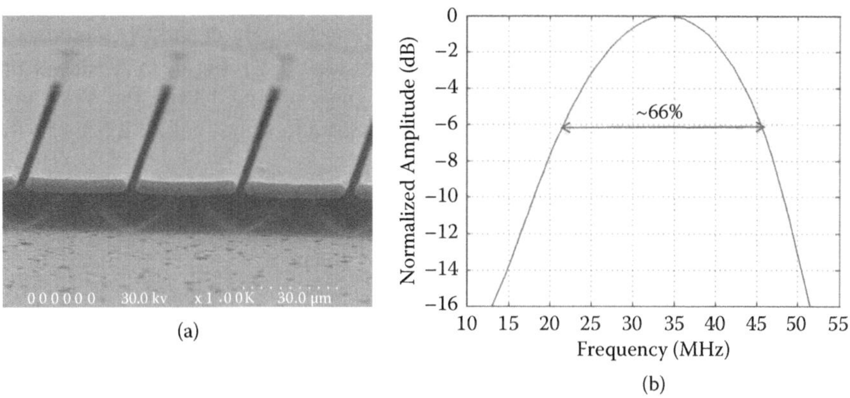

FIGURE 5.20 The SEM image of the thin-film transducer array (a) and its frequency spectrum (b).

bandwidth of 66% at 6 dB points. The capacitance of the 30 μm-wide transducer element is 145.1 pF, which indicates a dielectric constant of ~1000 at 1 kHz (as high as 1500) along with a low dielectric loss (<4%). Thus, the transducer appears to be a pure capacitance load for the preamplifier in the transceiver chip.

5.4.6.3 Pulse-Echo Experiments

The ultrasound signal acquisition experiments were conducted using the thin-film transducer with the transceiver chip. Figure 5.21 illustrates the pitch–catch mode experimental setup. The stainless steel target object was located at a distance of about

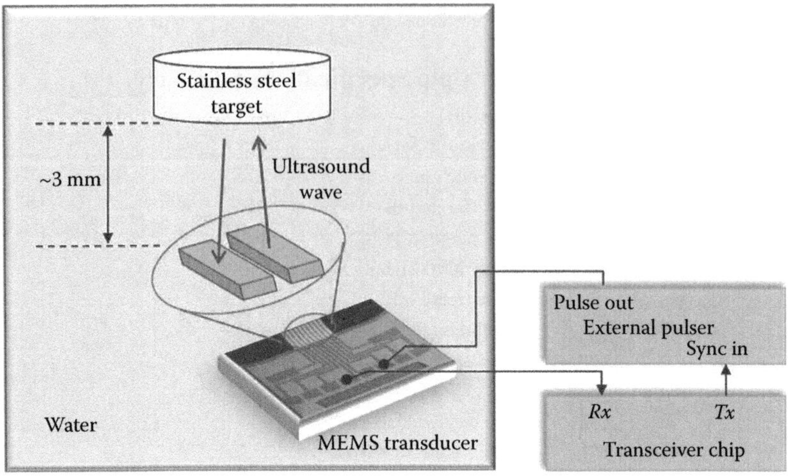

FIGURE 5.21 Pitch–catch mode experimental setup.

3 mm away from the transducers in the water tank. A 50 MHz transmit pulse sent to the thin-film transducers from the transceiver chip via an external pulser allowed an increase of acoustic energy. The adjacent transducer in the same array received the reflected signals; then, the transceiver chip amplified the received signals.

The gain of the preamplifier is set to 14 dB, and the gain of the VGA increased from 0 to 20 dB using varied control signals (0.15–1.0 V). Figure 5.22 shows the amplified and time-compensated ultrasound signals obtained from the VGA output using the thin-film transducer. The high-amplitude signal before 2.5 μs in the

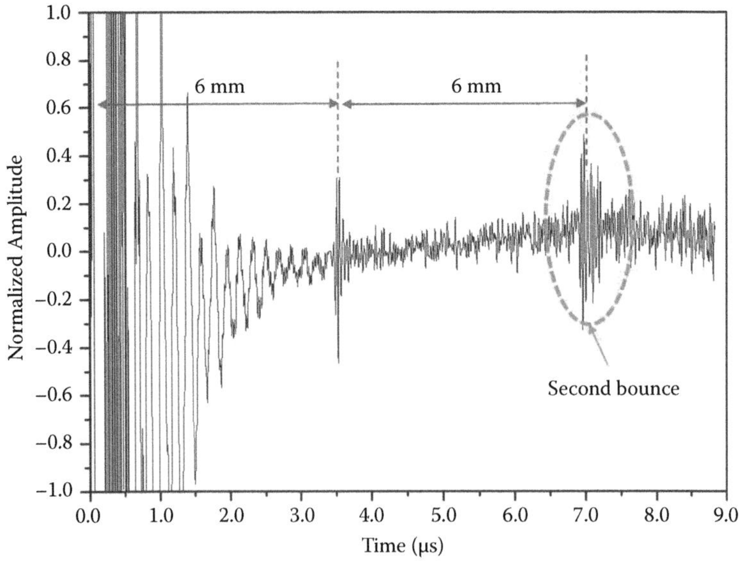

FIGURE 5.22 Thin-film transducer array pitch–catch mode test results.

figure is from cross talk with a transmit pulse. The first peak of the detected ultrasound wave appeared around 3.5 μs, which is the first echo signal; the second peaks, around 7 μs, underwent multiple bounces. The second peaks, amplified by the VGA, compensated for the attenuation in the water. Notably, the amplitude of the second peaks is similar to that of the first peak due to the increasing gain over the time.

5.5 CONCLUSION

This chapter explains the ultrasound imaging fundamentals and system considerations for developing a portable high-frequency ultrasound imaging system. The low-voltage transducer is crucial for developing a portable, ultra-compact ultrasound imaging system, because it enables the transducer to be placed with close-coupled ultrasound front-end electronics without using any expensive coaxial cables. Thus, reasonably, some cost reductions will accrue. Also, the fully integrated ultrasound transceiver chip with the shared ADC architecture is an effective solution for the portable imaging systems. It greatly decreases system size and power consumption, compared to conventional DBF ultrasound imaging systems currently marketed.

This chapter also introduces the Penn State portable ultrasound imaging system as an example of existing portable high-frequency ultrasound imaging systems. The Penn State ultrasound imaging system consists of low-voltage-operated thin-film transducer array and a fully integrated custom-designed CMOS transceiver chip. A 16 channel ultrasound receiver is shared with an A/D converter and a 3 Kb SRAM. The chip also makes it feasible for the transducers to be fabricated on the same package or board with the chip, and anticipates more cost and size reduction. Initial pulse-echo experiments using the imaging system were performed and the experimental results demonstrate the shared ADC architecture and the transceiver chip components designs.

REFERENCES

1. F.S. Foster, C.J. Pavlin, J.A. Harasiewicz, D. A. Christopher, and D.H. Turnbull, Advances in ultrasound biomicroscopy, *Ultrasound in Medicine and Biology*, 26(1):1–27, 2000.
2. P.A. Payne, J.V. Hatfield, A.D. Armitage, Q.X. Chen, P.J. Hicks, and N. Scales, Integrated ultrasound transducers, Proceedings of the IEEE Ultrasonic Symposium, Vol. 3, 1994, pp. 1523–1526.
3. R. Reeder and C. Petersen, The AD9271—A revolutionary solution for portable ultrasound, 2007 [Online]. http://www.analog.com/library/analogdialogue/archives/41-07/ultrasound.html Access date: 26-3-2014]
4. W.C. Black, Jr. and D.N. Stephens, CMOS chip for invasive ultrasound imaging, *IEEE Journal of Solid-State Circuits*, 29:11, 1994.
5. J.V. Hatfield, P.A. Payne, N.R. Scales, A.D. Armitage, and P.J. Hicks, Transmit and receive ASICs for an ultrasound imaging multi-element array transducer, IEEE Colloquium on ASICs for Measurement Systems, 1994.
6. I.O. Wygant, D.T. Yeh, X. Zhuang, S. Vaithilingam, A. Nikoozadeh, O. Oralkan, A. SanliErgun, G.G. Yaralioglu, and B.T. Khuri-Yakub, Integrated ultrasound imaging systems based on capacitive micromachined ultrasonic transducer arrays, *2005 IEEE Sensors*, 2005.

7. J. Johansson, M. Gustafsson, and J. Delsing, Ultra-low power transmit/receive ASIC for battery operated ultrasound measurement systems, *Sensors and Acturators A: Physical*, 125:317–328, 2006.
8. M.I. Fuller, E.V. Brush, M.D.C. Eames, T.N. Blalock, J.A. Hossack, and W.F. Walker, The sonic window: Second generation prototype of low-cost, fully-integrated, pocket-sized medical ultrasound device, *2005 IEEE Ultrasonics Symposium*, 2005, pp. 273–276.
9. I. Kim, H. Kim, F. Griggio, R.L. Tutwiler, T.N. Jackson, and S. Trolier-McKinstry, CMOS Ultrasound transceiver chip for high resolution ultrasonic imaging systems, *IEEE Transactions on Biomedical Circuits and Systems*, 3(5):293–303, 2009.
10. T.L. Szabo, *Wave Scattering and Imaging, Diagnostic Ultrasound Imaging: Inside Out*, Burlington, MA: Elsevier, 2004, pp. 213–242.
11. C.J. Pavlin and F.S. Foster, *Ultrasound Biomicroscopy of the Eye*, New York: Springer-Verlag, 1994.
12. M.E. Schafer and P.A. Lewin, The influence of front-end hardware on digital ultrasonic imaging, *IEEE Transactions on Sonics and Ultrasonics*, SU-31(4):295–306, 1984.
13. P.N.T. Wells, *Advances in Ultrasound Techniques and Instrumentation*, New York: Churchill Livingstone, 1993.
14. M. Karaman, E. Kolagasioglu, A. Atalar, A VLSI receive beamformer for digital ultrasound imaging, *IEEE International Conference on Acoustics, Speech, and Signal Processing,* San Francisco, CA, 1992, vol. 5, pp. 657-660.
15. A. Kassem, J. Wang, A. Khouas, M. Sawan, and M. Boukadoum, Pipelined sampled-delay focusing CMOS implementation for ultrasonic digital beamforming, *Proceedings of the 3rd IEEE Workshop on SoC for Real-time Application,* 2003, pp. 247–250.
16. I.G. Mina, H. Kim, I. Kim, S.K. Park, K. Choi, T.N. Jackson, R.L. Tutwiler, and S. Trolier-McKinstry, High frequency piezoelectric MEMS ultrasound transducers, *IEEE Transactions on Ultrasonics, Ferroelectrics, and Frequency Control*, 54(12):2422–2430, 2007.
17. S. Triger, J. Wallace, J.-F. Saillant, S. Cochran, and D.R.S. Cumming, MOSAIC: An integrated ultrasonic 2D array system, *2007 IEEE Ultrasonics Symposium,* New York, 2007.
18. B. Murmann, ADC Performance Survey 1997-2014, [Online]. Available: http://www.stanford.edu/~murmann/adcsurvey.html. Access date: 26-3-2014.
19. B. Murmann, A/D converter trends: Power dissipation, scaling and digitally assisted architectures, *IEEE 2008 Custom Integrated Circuits Conference (CICC),* San Jose, CA, September 21–24, 2008, pp. 105–112.
20. A.C. Kak and K.A. Dines, Signal processing of broad-band pulsed ultrasound: Measurement of attenuation of soft biological tissues, *IEEE Transactions on Biomedical Engineering*, BME-25:321–344, 1978.
21. H.B. Meire and P. Farrant, *Basic Ultrasound*, Chichester, UK: John Wiley & Sons, 1995.
22. R.J. Baker, *Data Converter SNR, in CMOS Mixed-Signal Circuit Design*, Vol. 2, Piscataway, NJ: IEEE Press, 2002, pp. 63–148.
23. B. Razavi, *Differential Amplifiers, in Design of Analog CMOS Integrated Circuits*, New York: McGraw-Hill, 2001, pp. 100–132.
24. C. Wu, C. Liu, and S. Liu, A 2GHz CMOS variable-gain amplifier with 50 dB linear-in-magnitude controlled gain range for 10GBase-LX4 ethernet, *ISSCC* 2004, Vol. 1, pp. 484–541.
25. C.E. Shannon, Communication in the presence of noise, *Proceedings Institute of Radio Engineers,* 37(1):10–21, 1949.
26. J. Yoo, D. Lee, K. Choi, and A. Tangle, Future-ready ultrafast 8-Bit CMOS ADC for system-on-chip applications, *14th Annual IEEE International ASIC/SOC Conference,* Arlington, VA, 2001, pp. 455–459.

27. J. Yoo, K. Choi, and D. Lee, Comparator generation and selection for highly linear CMOS flash analog-to-digital converter, *Journal of Analog Integrated Circuits and Signal Processing*, 35:179–187, 2003.
28. I. Kim, J. Yoo, J.-S. Kim, and K. Choi, Highly efficient comparator design automation for TIQ flash A/D converter, *IEICE Transactions on Fundamentals*, E91-A, 12:3415–3422, 2008.
29. UC Berkeley Device Group, BSIM, 2013 [Online]. Available: http://www-device.eecs.berkeley.edu/bsim/ Access date: 26-3-2014.
30. J.H. Kim, T.K. Song, and S.B. Park, Pipeline sampled-delay focusing in ultrasound imaging systems, *Journal of Ultrasonic Imaging*, 9:75–91, 1987.

Section 2

Information Processing and Implementation

6 Automated Blood Smear Analysis for Mobile Malaria Diagnosis

John A. Quinn, Alfred Andama, Ian Munabi, and Fred N. Kiwanuka

CONTENTS

6.1 INTRODUCTION

The gold standard test for malaria is the hundred-year-old method of preparing a blood smear on a glass slide, staining it, and examining it under a microscope to look for the parasite genus *Plasmodium*. While several rapid diagnostic tests are also currently available, they still have shortcomings compared to microscopic analysis [18]. In the regions worst affected by malaria, reliable diagnoses are often difficult to obtain, and treatment is routinely prescribed based only on symptoms. Accurate diagnosis is clearly important, since false negatives can be fatal and false positives lead to increased drug resistance, unnecessary economic burden, and possibly the failure to treat diseases with similar early symptoms such as meningitis or typhoid.

The scale of the problem is huge: annually there are 300–500 million cases of acute malaria illness of which 1.1–2.7 million are fatal, most fatalities being among children under the age of five [27,21,22].

The lack of access to diagnosis in developing countries is largely due to a shortage of expertise, with a shortage of equipment being a secondary factor. For example, a recent survey carried out in Uganda [34] found 50% of rural health centers to have microscopes, but only 17% had laboratory technicians with the training necessary to use them for malaria diagnosis. Even where a microscopist is available, they are often oversubscribed and cannot spend long enough examining each sample to give a confident diagnosis.

This situation has prompted an increasing interest in finding technological solutions to carrying out the diagnosis automatically with computer vision methods, taking advantage of existing equipment and compensating for the shortage of human expertise. In particular, image processing and computer vision techniques can be used to identify parasites in blood smear images captured through a standard microscope. Given sufficient training data, the algorithms used in other medical imaging problems or computer vision tasks such as face detection can be applied to recognize plasmodia. Some studies have looked further at classifying the species and life cycle stage of parasites.

Apart from the idea of using blood smear images captured directly from a microscope, there is a great deal of attention currently on other forms of point-of-care diagnosis for malaria. Some of these are reviewed in Section 6.2, and include methods based on fluorescence imaging or flow cytometry, for example. While these methods may be promising in the future, there is still value in diagnosis based on image processing currently, for the following reasons:

- Image processing methods can be used when we do not wish to remove human experts from the diagnostic process completely, but rather to offer decision support. In this case, we might display to a technician (either on site, or remotely) the regions in blood smear images which seem most indicative of plasmodium, and allow the technician to make the final judgment. This could improve the efficacy of technicians by helping to triage their attention, or make remote diagnosis over a network connection more feasible.
- When mobile devices are used for imaging and processing, we can take advantage of existing hardware. Both microscopes and camera phones are common in most malaria-affected countries. Hence, the only new hardware necessary to combine them is an adapter to mount the phone onto the microscope eyepiece or trinocular tube, which is relatively inexpensive. There have also been recent advances in low-cost microscopy using simple optical components attached to mobile devices [6,33].
- Several other tests can be carried out with the same images, for example cell counts or detection of other hemoparasites. Malaria diagnosis might be just one element of a suite of diagnostic software running on the same system. In principle, any microscopic test could be automated with the same imaging hardware given sufficient training examples.

The rest of the chapter is organized as follows. First we review existing work on point-of-care diagnosis for malaria, and the standard practice for malaria diagnosis. We then describe a typical image capture setup, including experiments with 3D-printed phone adapters. Next, we describe methodology for extracting statistical image features, and application of learning algorithms to carry out malaria diagnosis as an object detection problem. Finally, we provide some quantification of the accuracy of the system, and conclude with a discussion of current issues and future directions.

6.2 CONVENTIONAL MICROSCOPIC DIAGNOSIS OF MALARIA

The fundamental goal of malaria diagnosis is to demonstrate the presence of *Plasmodium* before antimalarial drugs are used. Presumptive diagnosis from symptoms alone has poor accuracy and can lead to overdiagnosis of malaria, with resultant poor management of nonmalarial febrile illnesses and wastage of antimalarial drugs [19]. Definitive diagnosis of malaria infection is still based on finding malaria parasites microscopically in stained blood films.

In thin films the red blood cells are fixed so the morphology of the parasitized cells can be seen. Species identification can be made, based on the size and shape of the various stages of the parasite and the presence of stippling (i.e., bright red dots) and fimbriation (i.e., ragged ends). However, malaria parasites may be missed on a thin blood film when there is a low parasitemia. Therefore, examination of a thick blood smear, which is 20–40 times more sensitive than thin smears for screening of plasmodium parasites, with a detection limit of 10–50 trophozoites/μL is recommended [28]. In this process, the red blood cells are lysed and diagnosis is based on the appearance of the parasites which tend to be more compact and denser than in thin films. Since the thick smear is approximately 6–20 times as thick as a single layer of red blood cells, this results in a larger volume of blood being examined.

A group of dyes known as *Romanowsky stains* are a series of blue/red stains where the blue (methylene blue) binds to acidic substances and the red (eosin) binds to neutral or basic substances in cells. Examples of such stains include Field's A and B, Giemsa, Leishman, and Wright's stain. Developed in the 1800s by the Russian physician Romanowsky, these stains have similar basic components but differ from each other according to simple modifications.

While Leishman's stain (1901) undoubtedly gives the best results in a thin film, Giemsa stain (1902) has proved to be the best all-round stain for the routine diagnosis of malaria. It has the disadvantage of being relatively expensive, but this is outweighed by its stability over time and its consistent staining quality over a wide range of temperatures. The detection threshold in Giemsa-stained thick blood film has been estimated to be 4–20 parasites/μL [20]. Under field conditions, a threshold of about 50–100 parasites/μL blood is more realistic [16]. However, in remote settings with less skilled microscopists and poor equipment, a still higher threshold is likely.

The method preferred for staining thick blood smears in countries such as Uganda is Field's stain, particularly because it is more rapid than the alternatives. This stain is made of two components: Field's A is a buffered solution of azure dye and Field's B is a buffered solution of eosin. These stains are supplied ready to use by the manufacturer, and have advantages of being inexpensive, simple to use, economical, and have short staining time compared to other methods. However there are also disadvantages with Field's stain, especially in under-resourced health centers in which the stain might be used. Poor blood film preparations often result in the generation of artifacts commonly mistaken for malaria parasites, such as bacteria, fungi, stain precipitation, and dirt and cell debris. These can frequently cause false positive readings [11].

6.2.1 Practical Difficulties in Under-Resourced Health Facilities

The procedure of staining with Field's A and B involves dipping the slide into the solution. This normally requires pouring the stains in couplin jars, which ideally should have lids, and water between them. These solutions are supposed to be prepared fresh each day for optimum potency, or kept tightly closed and filtered every morning. However, in resource constrained settings—under which the majority of health facilities in Uganda fall—these jars could be kept for weeks, and the stains rarely filtered. Frequent opening of these jars results in evaporation of methanol, which then results into precipitation artifacts. Contamination can also result from stain or water carry-over from one jar to the other (dilution). Bacterial contamination can originate from frequent opening of the jars or be introduced from dirty slides, and if not filtered regularly can result into false positive reporting as bacterial cells could be confused with malaria parasites.

Another contributing factor to poor microscopy performance is excessive workload, which is a problem when there is a shortage of staff with sufficient expertise. Sensitivity is directly related to the time available to examine blood films and therefore decreases when the number of slides exceeds the workload capacity of the microscopist, and this becomes more pronounced if the microscopist has responsibilities for diagnosing other diseases.

The time required to read an individual malaria slide depends on several factors, including the quality of microscope and immersion oil used, the skill of the microscopist, slide positivity rate (SPR), and parasite density. The time taken to declare a slide positive or negative differs considerably. A strongly positive thick film can be examined more quickly than a weak positive or more still a negative film. Another significant factor is the additional time required for species differentiation, where this is clinically important. Species identification is best done on a thin smear, but in low parasite density is extremely time-consuming.

During the malaria eradication era, the World Health Organization (WHO) recommended that a single technician can satisfactorily read 60–75 slides per day. More recently, this has been considered unrealistic as a standard since the functions and roles of microscopists in malaria control are different today. Based on the Ugandan situation, the Malaria Control Programme together with the Malaria Consortium have recommended 25–40 slides per day, each covering about 200 microscopic fields from a standard thick smear using x100 objective. This should take 5 to 10 minutes on average to declare a smear negative [4]. However, according to our personal experience, even after examining 20 consecutive slides, fatigue becomes an issue and concentration tends to weaken.

Perhaps the most important constraint for microscopy-based diagnosis in the developing world, however, is the frequent absence altogether of laboratory technicians from health facilities in rural areas. In Uganda, with only 34% of the laboratory staff positions occupied, the absence of this cadre of staff has been associated with higher costs of diagnostics based on microscopy in comparison with those based on rapid diagnostic tests (RDTs) [5,36]. The absence of human resources for health is a major problem in sub-Saharan Africa, and one which gets worse in the lower health units which are commonly the first point of contact for patients.

6.3 ALTERNATIVE DIAGNOSIS METHODS

The absence of human resource for performing the diagnosis of malaria in these settings is one of the reasons for the development of alternatives methods of diagnosis. This includes the recent development of several RDTs for malaria, methods for automating the microscopic examination with image processing, and other forms of diagnosis. In this section we review alternatives to the conventional diagnosis methods.

6.3.1 Rapid Diagnostic Tests

Rapid diagnostic tests (RDTs) for malaria have been a great success in reducing the disease burden following the change in policy by WHO [12,35]. RDTs, based on testing for antigens produced by the immune system in response to plasmodium, have high sensitivity for parasite concentrations of over 500/μL. For smaller concentrations the sensitivity of RDTs becomes too low to be used reliably, however [36]. Test results are usually available in 5 to 20 minutes, do not require capital investment, electricity, or extensive training for laboratory staff, although individual tests are more expensive with RDTs than microscopic analysis [5].

Apart from the issues of inadequate sensitivity for low parasite concentrations, there are other concerns about the discriminative effectiveness of RDTs in specific situations. These include frequent false positive results in areas of low transmission [2] and false negatives for individuals with asymptomatic infections or multiple organism infestations [14]. Overall, RDTs are successful in a number of situations, but the gold standard for diagnosis for malaria remains the microscope—especially in those instances such as treatment failures or low parasitemia where RDTs will not work [1,13].

6.3.2 Related Work in Computer Vision Diagnostics

A number of studies have looked at image processing and computer vision methodology for automated diagnosis of malaria from blood smears. In vision terms this is an object detection problem, and some previous work is reviewed in [31]. There has also been work in comparing these methods with other forms of diagnosis [3]. Reference [24] uses neural networks with morphological features to identify red blood cells and possible parasites present on a microscopic slide. The results obtained with this technique were 85% recall and 81% precision using a set of 350 images containing 950 objects. In [30] a distance weighted k-nearest neighbor classifier was trained with features extracted by use of a Bayesian pixel classifier which was used to mark the stained pixels. The results achieved by this method were 74% recall and 88% precision.

Color space and morphological heuristics were employed to segment red blood cells and parasites by using an optimal saturation threshold [15] using a set of 55 images. Multi-class parasite identification, attempting to classify the type and life cycle stage of detected parasites has also been attempted [32].

All the vision systems mentioned operate on images of thin blood films, a single layer of blood cells with red blood cell matter preserved. Thick blood film images, which are prepared in such a way that red blood cell matter is destroyed and DNA material is stained, are more commonly used in the developing world as they are more sensitive. This makes diagnosis possible even with very low parasitemia, although typing of parasites is difficult with this type of sample as shape information is not as well preserved. Furthermore, the samples used in these previous studies were prepared under ideal conditions, with high quality slide preparation and imaging equipment. In the experiments described here, we use thick film images collected under field conditions.

6.4 BLOOD SMEAR IMAGE CAPTURE AND ANNOTATION

In order to automate the process of parasite detection, we first consider two different methods for capturing images of blood smears under a microscope: using a dedicated microscope camera, or using the camera of a mobile device such as a smartphone. For the latter method, we investigated the potential of 3D printing for producing low-cost adapters with which to mount a phone directly on the eyepiece of the microscope. The promise of this type of 3D printing approach is that customized adapters could in principle be made on demand for any combination of camera phone and microscope, as long as the geometry of the phone and the eyepiece diameter of the microscope eyepiece are known. Figure 6.1 (top) shows the design of our prototype adapter for attaching a ZTE Blade low cost Android smartphone to a Brunel SP150 microscope. Combining the imaging and computation on a single device, particularly a device already widely available even in malaria-endemic regions, would clearly make the system quite practical to deploy. Figure 6.1 (bottom) shows the printed adapter on one eyepiece, and a Motic MC1000 microscope camera on the other eyepiece.

Samples of the images taken from the camera phone and the dedicated microscope camera are shown in Figure 6.2. The image from the camera phone is clear, but has a wider field of view than the dedicated microscope camera. A single parasite is about 20 pixels across in the Motic image, but only around 8 pixels across in the image taken with the phone camera. We concluded that the phone imaging setup is a promising, low cost method for capturing blood film images for diagnosis, but that more work is needed on building extra magnification into such adapters in order to obtain a sufficient level of detail on plasmodium objects. The experiments described in the following parts of this chapter all use images from the Motic camera.

Sets of images were taken of thick blood smears with Field's stain from 133 individuals, using 1000x magnification with an oil immersion objective lens. After eliminating images which were out of focus, had motion artifacts from movement of the microscope stage during image capture, or were hyperparasitemic to the extent that it would be impractical to confidently label every parasite in the image, we were left with a set of 2703 images.

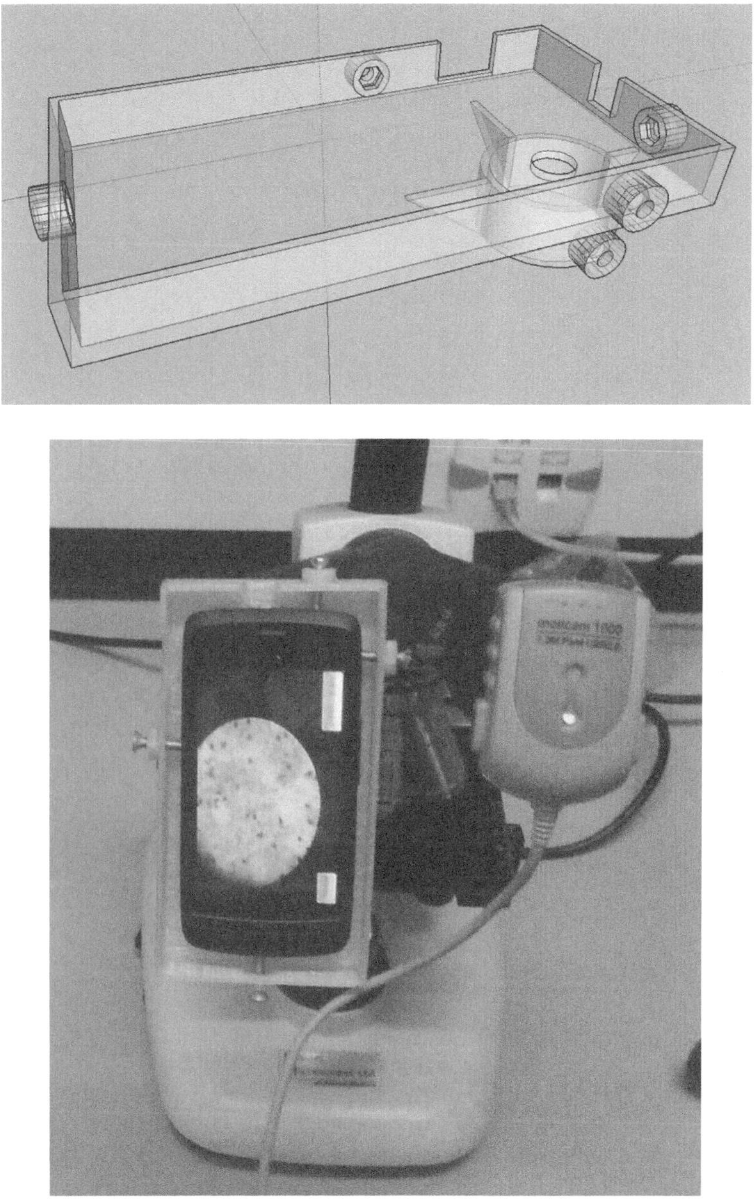

FIGURE 6.1 3D-printable design for smartphone adapter (top). Printed phone adapter and Motic camera mounted on microscope (bottom).

6.4.1 Annotation

In order to train and test the automated diagnosis system, it was necessary to annotate each of these images with the bounding boxes around each parasite. Bounding boxes were annotated on the captured images using labeling software developed

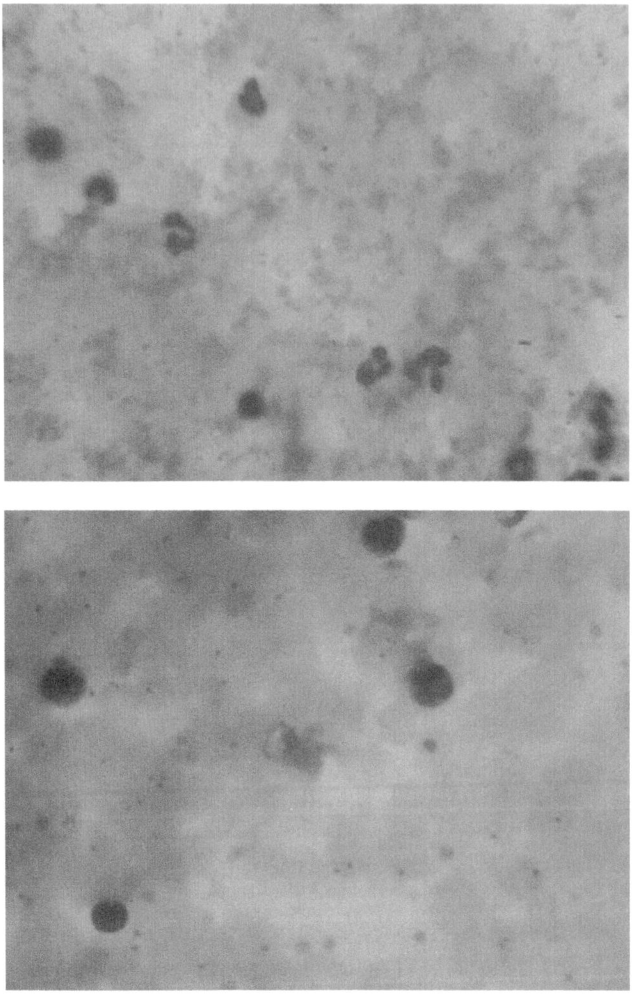

FIGURE 6.2 Image from camera-phone (top), and image from Motic camera (bottom).

for the PASCAL Visual Object Classes challenge [7]. A team of four experienced laboratory technicians used this software to indicate the position of every object they judged to be a parasite. Sample annotations are shown in Figure 6.3 (top). In this way the coordinates of 50,255 parasites were recorded within the set of captured images.

6.5 AUTOMATED DIAGNOSIS

We split up each image into overlapping patches, and assigned each patch a label of 0 or 1, depending on whether the center of a parasite bounding box was within that patch. Each 1024×768 image was split into 475 overlapping patches, each of size 50×50 pixels. Given this labeled set of image patches, we can pose the plasmodium detection task as a classification problem. To illustrate the nature of this problem,

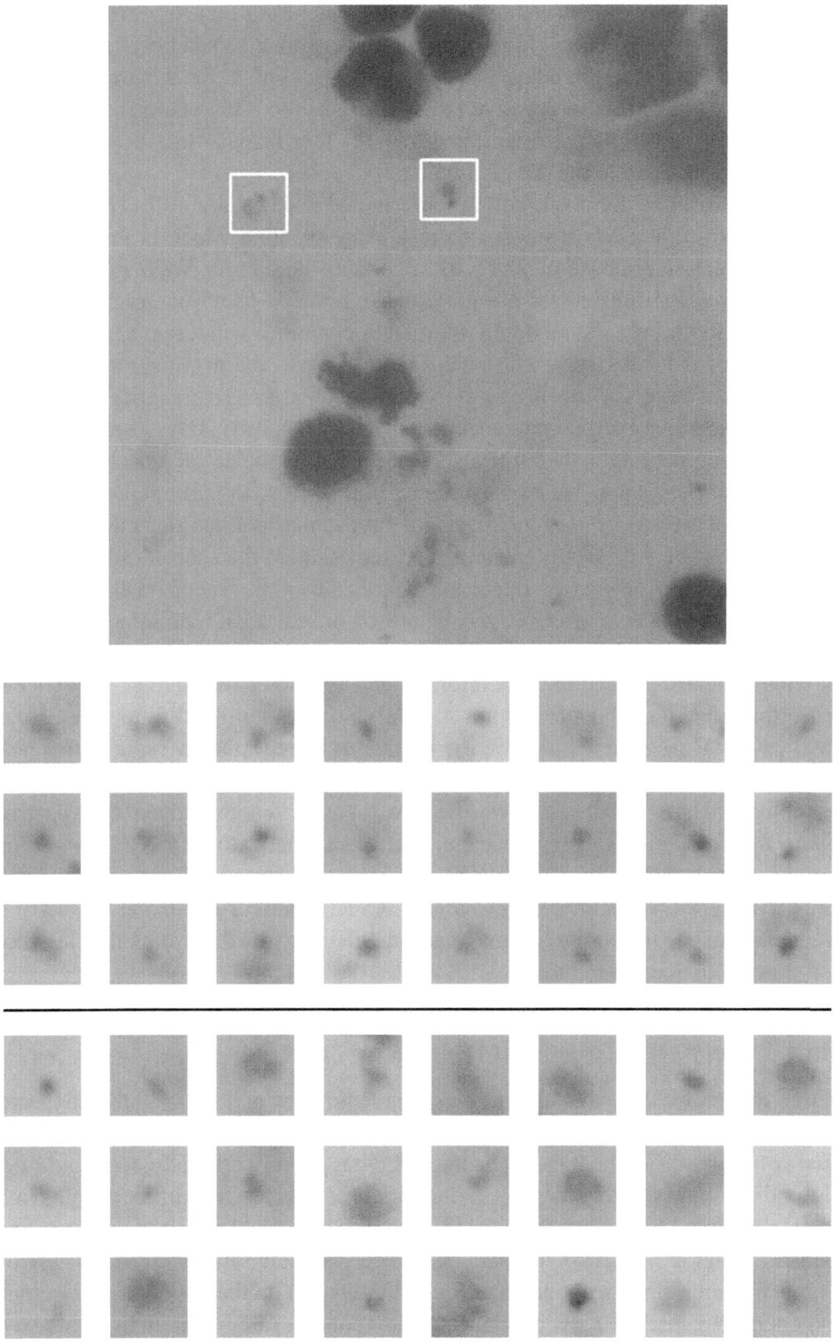

FIGURE 6.3 Bounding boxes around parasites annotated on a training image (top). Sample image patches close to the decision boundary, positive cases at the top and negative cases at the bottom (bottom).

and its difficulties, we show examples of image patches in Figure 6.3 (bottom). The patches in the upper section of the figure all have a positive label (i.e., they contain the center of a parasite bounding box as specified by one of the expert annotators). The lower patches all have negative labels (i.e., they do not contain the center of a bounding box), but contain artifacts, platelets, or other shapes which might appear to a classifier to be close to the decision boundary.

The raw form of the pixel data in these image patches is not directly very useful for classification. We instead require a representation which is invariant with respect to rotation, translation, and constant offsets in intensity. We may also require scale invariance if the images are not collected with a fixed magnification. Since the patches in the parasite recognition problem contain plasmodium against a background of normal cell matter, it also helps in this case to engineer features with some concept of an "object." This is common in biomedical imaging applications, where we wish to segment images into objects such as organs, cells, and so on.

Feature engineering is therefore a significant step in the development of the automated diagnosis system. We have two aims in this: first, to find a representation of the data which leads to good performance on the plasmodium detection task, and second, to have a sufficiently general representation of the shapes in blood smear images that other objects of interest—such as different hemoparasites, or white blood cells—could also be effectively identified in future with the same platform.

The plasmodium detection problem primarily concerns the shape of objects in the input patches. In general color information can also be useful (e.g., with Giemsa or Leishman stains), though it is not so informative using blood films treated with Field's stain. Hence the features we use for this task are statistical representations of the shapes found in the image patches, and for all feature extraction we first convert the color patches to grayscale. We use two types of features: those derived from *connected components*, using concepts from mathematical morphology, and those derived from calculating moments of the patches thresholded at multiple levels. These two types of features are explained in Sections 6.5.1 and 6.5.2, respectively. We then conclude the automated diagnosis methodology by describing the classification process in Section 6.5.3.

6.5.1 Connected Component Features

In this section we describe features based on regions, which are spatially connected sets of pixels that have some property in common such as similar grey level, and are used to define disjoint image segments. Regions, if properly defined, should correspond to objects. However, proper definition of regions is a difficult problem in image analysis. One approach to this problem, which has been used extensively in medical imaging, is a class of operators called connected filters [26,10]. These are a family of morphological operators [9] that are based on the notion of connectivity and operate by interacting with connected components rather than individual pixels. Connectivity describes the way pixels are grouped to form connected components or flat zones in gray scale.

To calculate shape features for an image patch in this way, we first thresholded the image at each gray level. Connectivity openings [23] were used to calculate all the

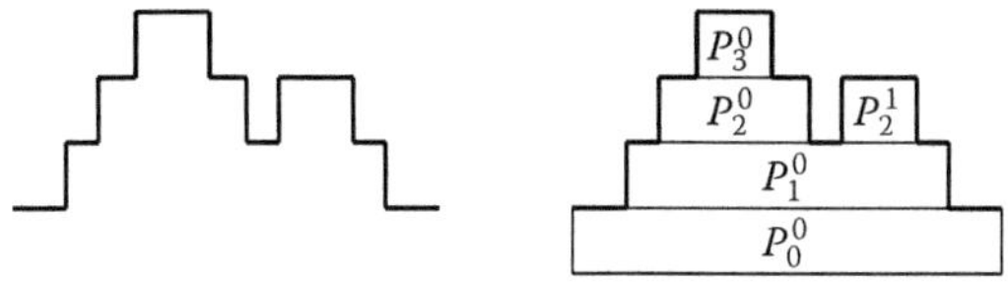

FIGURE 6.4 A 1D signal f (left), and the corresponding peak components (right).

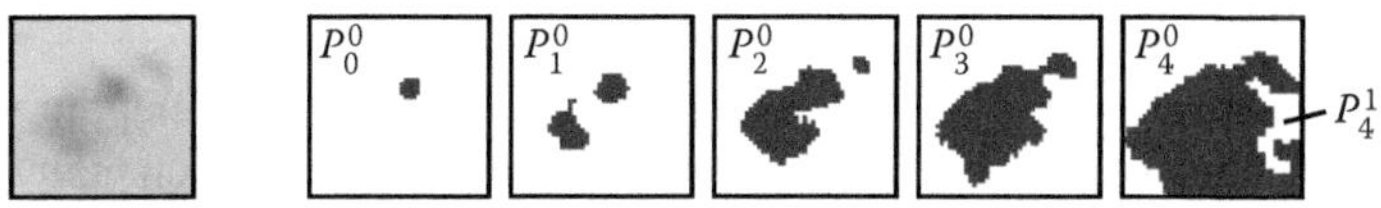

FIGURE 6.5 Sample grayscale patch containing a parasite (left), and connected peak components—indicated as white regions—at different threshold levels (right).

components in each thresholded image. These are known as *peak components* and denoted as P_h^k for gray level h and index k. This is illustrated in Figure 6.4 for a 1D example, and Figure 6.5 for an example with an image patch containing a parasite. The peak components were used to construct a max tree [25], which is a data structure designed for morphological image processing in order to efficiently compute features or attributes of the connected components. The max tree makes it possible to compute a large number of shape attributes for each of its nodes, and classification can then be based on these computed properties.

We computed several common morphological features for the connected components of every image patch, then used feature selection to narrow these down to five features most informative for the parasite detection task. These selected features are as follows:

- Perimeter
- Moment of Inertia
- Elongation: Inertia/Area^2
- Jaggedness: (Area × Perimeter^2)/($8\pi^2$ × Inertia)
- Maximum λ: Maximum child gray level – current gray level

Our aim was to compute standardized feature vectors for each patch in an image. Because the number of components on a single patch is variable, we summarized the shape information by traversing the max tree and calculating the percentile distribution of every attribute. For the five features above, we calculated the 25th, 50th, 75th percentiles, and the minimum and maximum values. Therefore we obtained a 25-dimensional feature vector for each image patch.

6.5.2 Moment Features

An additional set of features was obtained by thresholding each patch at five different levels between the minimum and maximum pixel value. For each of the binary images returned by the threshold operation, we calculated many standard moment statistics [29] and used feature selection methods on training data to find those which were most discriminative with respect to the patch label. In this way, we selected the moment m_{00}, the central moments μ_{11}, μ_{20}, μ_{02}, and Hu moments h_0, h_1, h_2. These seven statistics, calculated for five different thresholded versions of the patch, therefore provided an additional 35 features for each patch. These features were appended to those calculated as described in the previous section.

6.5.3 Classification

The Extremely Randomized Trees classifier [8] was used to learn a mapping between features and patch labels. This is a type of ensemble method, in which many decision trees are learned by selecting thresholds at random and retaining the trees which give good classification performance. Its advantages for this application, as well as good discriminative performance, are that it is fast and memory-efficient to evaluate at test time. This is useful for situations where classification is to be carried out on a mobile device with limited computational resources. An ensemble of 250 trees, with a maximum tree depth of five was used.

6.6 EVALUATION

The classifier was trained on 75% of the labeled data (2027 images, containing 37,550 patches annotated as containing parasites), and tested on the remaining 25% (676 images, containing 16,312 patches annotated as containing parasites). Figure 6.6 provides an illustration of the classifier output on test data, showing sample image patches grouped by classification probability.

The receiver operating characteristic (ROC) curve is shown in Figure 6.7 (top), and the area under the curve (AUC) of 0.97 indicates that the classifier is effective at distinguishing positive and negative patches. Note that this is the performance at determining whether individual image patches contain parasites, not the performance at classifying all the image data from a single patient. If there are one or more positive patches within the set of images from an individual sample, then that sample is considered infected. We

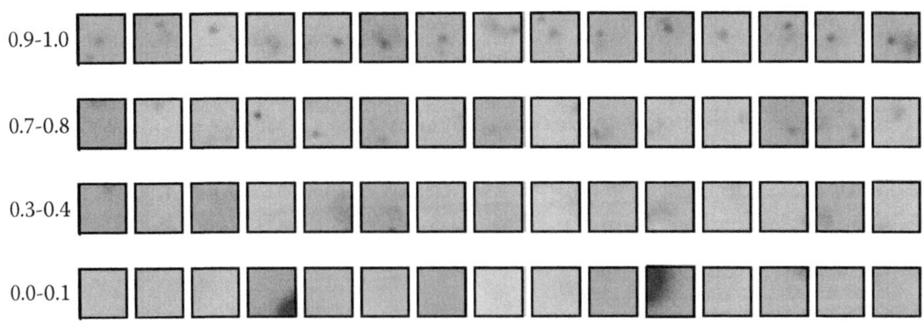

FIGURE 6.6 Sample patches in test images, arranged by the probability assigned by the classifier to each patch of its containing a parasite. The probability range of each row is indicated on the left, with the top row being patches confidently classified as positive cases, and the bottom row being confidently classified as negative cases.

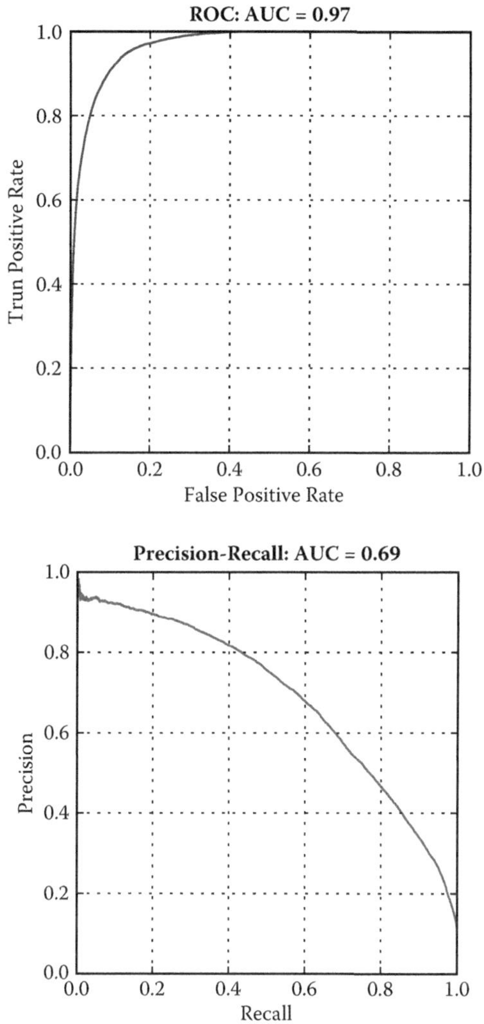

FIGURE 6.7 Receiver operating characteristics (top) and precision-recall curves for test data (bottom).

cannot give per-patient sensitivity and specificity results here, as nearly all of the blood smear images in our experiments were from malaria-infected individuals.

The precision-recall curve, shown in Figure 6.7 (bottom) shows the different trade-offs possible between increasing sensitivity and decreasing the false alarm rate. Note that this compares favorably to the performance of related methods for thin blood smear analysis in Section 6.3.2, given that thick blood smears are an order of magnitude more sensitive than thin blood smears. Therefore, if we choose a detection threshold that gives us precision of 90%, the corresponding recall of around 20% is still higher than any method using thin blood smears would be able to attain after analyzing the same number of fields of view. Figure 6.8 shows an example of

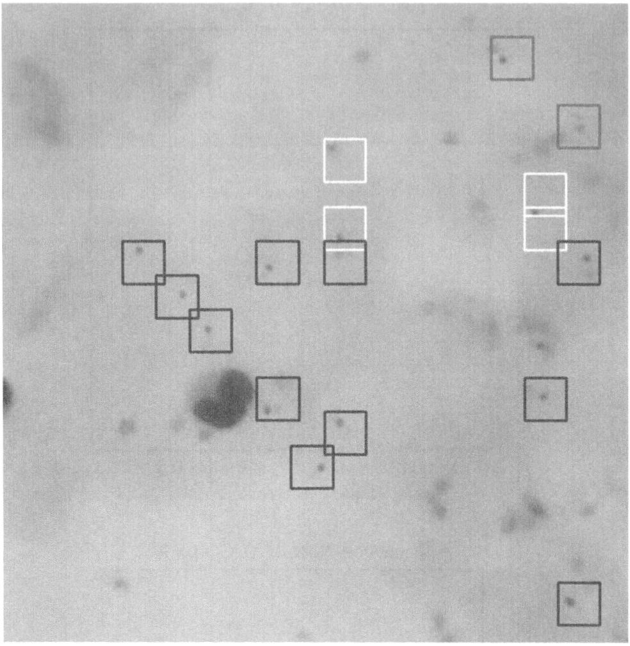

FIGURE 6.8 Sample detection output on part of a test image. Black squares indicate patches which were correctly classified as containing parasites (where the classifier gave a probability above a threshold of 0.8, and the patch label was positive), gray squares indicate false positives (classifier probability above threshold, but label negative) and white squares indicate false negatives (classifier probability below threshold, but label positive). By adjusting the classification threshold, different trade-offs are found between false positives and false negatives.

true positives, false positives and false negatives on a test image for one particular detection threshold.

From Figure 6.7 (bottom) we can see that if the system were to be used for entirely automated diagnosis, in order to have a false alarm rate below one in ten, the recall would be around one fifth of what an experienced laboratory technician would be able to achieve; that is, the minimum detectable concentration of parasites in the blood would be around five times higher for the automated system than for the human expert. This is better than a purely symptomatic diagnosis, but clearly has shortcomings in terms of sensitivity. An alternative way to use such a system, therefore, would be as a decision-making aid to a technician. The aim in this context is to process the images from the microscope in order to focus the technician's attention on only the objects within those images that most resemble plasmodium. For this, a different threshold with greater sensitivity would be appropriate. For example, we might require recall of 90%, giving a corresponding precision of 37%. That is, we would expect the system to detect nine of every ten parasites appearing in the images, but 63% of detections would be false alarms. This would be discriminative enough to considerably improve the throughput of a technician, who would only have to assess highlighted regions, rather than entire images.

The system was implemented in Python with scikit-learn* and opencv.† Feature extraction code was implemented in C for computational efficiency. Video of a netbook deployment operating in a clinical setting can be seen online.‡

6.7 DISCUSSION

In this chapter we have given a methodology for automated diagnosis of malaria from blood smear images, including image capture, feature extraction, and classification. The accuracy of the system currently makes it practical as a decision-making aid for laboratory technicians, by triaging attention to the parts of images most indicative of plasmodium. For fully automated diagnosis, in order to have a false alarm rate below 10%, the sensitivity would be around 20% of what a trained microscopist would be able to achieve with the same images. This is still likely to be more sensitive than an analysis based on thin blood smears, which has been the focus of most previous work on vision-based automated malaria diagnosis, and certainly more sensitive than rapid diagnostic tests.

A platform for the automation of diagnosis from blood smear images provides several interesting and useful directions for future work. A location-aware mobile device could look up its location on a risk map, in order to set a prior for diagnosis (discussed further in [17]). Automated diagnosis also provides a significant opportunity for data collection; if test results are stored centrally, then spatial patterns of malaria incidence could be inferred. Furthermore, the feature extraction and classification framework we have described is sufficiently general that a whole suite of diagnostic tests—e.g., for tuberculosis, worm infestations, or hemoparasites other than plasmodium—could feasibly be implemented using the same framework.

6.8 ACKNOWLEDGMENTS

This work was funded in part by a grant from Microsoft Research. Annotation of blood smear images was carried out by Alfred Andama, Vincent Wadda, Steven Ikodi, and Patrick Byanyima. 3D printing was done by Sandeep Patel and Kenan Pollack of OmusonoLabs, Kampala. Mark Everingham provided us with image annotation software.

REFERENCES

1. K. Abba, J.J. Deeks, P. Olliaro, C-M. Naing, S.M. Jackson, Y. Takwoingi, S. Donegan, and P. Garner. Rapid diagnostic tests for diagnosing uncomplicated *P. falciparum* malaria in endemic countries. *Cochrane Database Syst Rev*, 7, 2011.
2. L. Allen, J. Hatfield, G. DeVetten, J. Ho, and M. Manyama. Reducing malaria misdiagnosis: The importance of correctly interpreting Paracheck Pf. *BMC Infectious Diseases*, 11(1):308, 2011.

---

* Scikit-Learn (http://scikit-learn.org).
† OpenCV (http://opencv.org).
‡ AI-DEV: Artificial Intelligence in the Developing World (http://aidevmakerere.blogspot.com/2012/08/live-testing-of-computer-vision-malaria.html).

3. B.B. Andrade, A. Reis-Filho, A.M. Barros, S.M. Souza-Neto, L.L. Nogueira, K.F. Fukutani, E.P. Camargo, L.M.A. Camargo, A. Barral, A. Duarte, and M. Barral-Netto. Towards a precise test for malaria diagnosis in the Brazilian Amazon: Comparison among field microscopy, a rapid diagnostic test, nested PCR, and a computational expert system based on artificial neural networks. *Malaria Journal*, 9:117, 2010.
4. J. Bailey, J. Williams, B.J. Bain, J. Parker-Williams, and P.L. Chiodini. Guideline: The laboratory diagnosis of malaria. *British Journal of Haematology*, 163(5):573–580, 2013.
5. V. Batwala, P. Magnussen, K.S. Hansen, F. Nuwaha, et al. Cost-effectiveness of malaria microscopy and rapid diagnostic tests versus presumptive diagnosis: Implications for malaria control in Uganda. *Malaria Journal*, 10(1):372, 2011.
6. D.N. Breslauer, R.N. Maamari, N.A. Switz, W.A. Lam, and D.A. Fletcher. Mobile phone based clinical microscopy for global health applications. *PLoS One*, 4(7):e6320, 2009.
7. M. Everingham, L. Van Gool, C.K.I. Williams, J. Winn, and A. Zisserman. The PASCAL visual object classes (VOC) challenge. *International Journal of Computer Vision*, 88(2):303–338, 2010.
8. P. Geurts, D. Ernst, and L. Wehenkel. Extremely randomized trees. *Machine Learning*, 63(1):3–42, 2006.
9. H.J.A.M. Heijmans. *Morphological Image Operators*. Boston: Academic Press, 1994.
10. H.J.A.M. Heijmans. Connected morphological operators for binary images. *Computer Vision and Image Understanding*, 73:99–120, 1999.
11. B. Houwen. Blood film preparation and staining procedures. *Laboratory Hematology*, 6(1):1–7, 2000.
12. D.S. Ishengoma, F. Francis, B.P. Mmbando, J.P.A. Lusingu, P. Magistrado, M. Alifrangis, T.G. Theander, I.C. Bygbjerg, and M.M. Lemnge. Accuracy of malaria rapid diagnostic tests in community studies and their impact on treatment of malaria in an area with declining malaria burden in north-eastern Tanzania. *Malaria Journal*, 10:176, 2011.
13. M. Kiggundu, S.L. Nsobya, M.R. Kamya, S. Filler, S. Nasr, G. Dorsey, and A. Yeka. Evaluation of a comprehensive refresher training program in malaria microscopy covering four districts of Uganda. *The American Journal of Tropical Medicine and Hygiene*. 84(5):820, 2011.
14. O.A. Koita, O.K. Doumbo, A. Ouattara, L.K. Tall, A. Konaré, M. Diakité, M. Diallo, I. Sagara, G.L. Masinde, S.N. Doumbo, et al. False-negative rapid diagnostic tests for malaria and deletion of the histidine-rich repeat region of the hrp2 gene. *The American Journal of Tropical Medicine and Hygiene*, 86(2):194–198, 2012.
15. V.V. Makkapati and R.M. Rao. Segmentation of malaria parasites in peripheral blood smear images. *IEEE International Conference on Acoustics, Speech and Signal Processing*, Taipei, April 19–24, 2009.
16. L.M. Milne, M.S. Kyi, P.L. Chiodini, and D.C. Warhurst. Accuracy of routine laboratory diagnosis of malaria in the United Kingdom. *Journal of Clinical Pathology*, 47(8):740–742, 1994.
17. M.G. Mubangizi, C. Ikae, A. Spiliopoulou, and J.A. Quinn. Coupling spatiotemporal disease modeling with diagnosis. In *Proceedings of the International Conference on Artificial Intelligence (AAAI)*, Toronto, July 22–26, 2012.
18. C.K. Murray, R.A. Gasser, A.J. Magill, and R.S. Miller. Update on rapid diagnostic testing for malaria. *Clinical Microbiology Reviews*, 21:97–110, 2008.
19. World Health Organization. Malaria light microscopy: Creating a culture of quality. In *Report of WHO SEARO/WPRO Workshop on Quality Assurance for Malaria Microscopy*, Geneva, 2005.
20. D. Payne. Use and limitations of light microscopy for diagnosing malaria at the primary health care level. *Bulletin of the World Health Organization*, 66(5):621, 1988.

21. M.E. Rafael, T. Taylor, A. Magill, Y-W Lim, F. Girosi, and R. Allan. Reducing the burden of childhood malaria in Africa. *Nature*, 444:39–48, 2006.
22. A. Roca-Feltrer, I. Carneiro, and J.R.M. Schellenberg. Estimates of the burden of malaria morbidity in Africa in children under the age of 5 years. *Tropical Medicine & International Health*, 13(6):771–783, 2008.
23. C. Ronse. Set-theoretical algebraic approaches to connectivity in continuous or digital spaces. *J. Math. Imag. Vis.*, 8:41–58, 1998.
24. N.E. Ross, C.J. Pritchard, D.M. Rubin, and A.G. Duse. Automated image processing method for the diagnosis and classification of malaria on thin blood smear. *Med Biol Eng Comput*, 44:427–436, 2006.
25. P. Salembier, A. Oliveras, and L. Garrido. Anti-extensive connected operators for image and sequence processing. *IEEE Trans. Image Proc.*, 7:555–570, 1998.
26. P. Salembier and J. Serra. Flat zones filtering, connected operators, and filters by reconstruction. *IEEE Trans. Image Proc.*, 4:1153–1160, 1995.
27. E.M. Samba. The burden of malaria in Africa. *Afr. Health*, 19(2):17, 1997.
28. N. Tangpukdee, C. Duangdee, P. Wilairatana, and S. Krudsood. Malaria diagnosis: A brief review. *The Korean Journal of Parasitology*, 47(2):93–102, 2009.
29. C.-H. Teh and R.T. Chin. On image analysis by the methods of moments. *IEEE Transactions on Pattern Analysis and Machine Intelligence,* 10(4):496–513, 1988.
30. F.B. Tek, A.G. Dempster, and I. Kale. Malaria parasite detection in peripheral blood images. *British Machine Vision Conference*, pp. 347–56, Edinburgh, September 4–7, 2006.
31. F.B. Tek, A.G. Dempster, and I. Kale. Computer vision for microscopy diagnosis of malaria. *Malaria Journal*, 8:153, 2009.
32. F.B. Tek, A.G. Dempster, and I. Kale. Parasite detection and identification for automated thin blood film malaria diagnosis. *Computer Vision and Image Understanding*, 114(1):21–32, 2010.
33. D. Tseng, O. Mudanyali, C. Oztoprak, S.O. Isikman, I. Sencan, O. Yaglidere, and A. Ozcan. Lensfree microscopy on a cellphone. *Lab on a Chip*, 10(14):1787–1792, 2010.
34. M. Tumwebaze. Evaluation of the capacity to appropriately diagnose and treat malaria at rural health centers in Kabarole District, Western Uganda. *Health Policy and Development*, 9(1):46–51, 2011.
35. H.A. Williams, L. Causer, E. Metta, A. Malila, T. O'Reilly, S. Abdulla, S.P. Kachur, and P.B. Bloland. Dispensary level pilot implementation of rapid diagnostic tests: An evaluation of RDT acceptance and usage by providers and patients–Tanzania, 2005. *Malaria Journal*, 7(1):239, 2008.
36. C. Wongsrichanalai, M.J. Barcus, S. Muth, A. Sutamihardja, and W.H. Wernsdorfer. A review of malaria diagnostic tools: Microscopy and rapid diagnostic test (RDT). *The American Journal of Tropical Medicine and Hygiene*, 77(6 Suppl):119–127, 2007.

7 Usability Engineering for Mobile Point-of-Care Devices

Grace Bartoo and Terese Bogucki

CONTENTS

7.1 INTRODUCTION

The application of mobile technologies to improve medicine at the point of care is quickly expanding. While there is a desire to increase the reach of health monitoring and diagnostics, designers and developers should consider the user and usability of these applications. Applying a thorough usability engineering process during product development can mean the difference between a medical device being widely adopted versus being subjected to a recall. Most people have had the experience of becoming frustrated with a product that was not as simple to use as desired or expected. These types of products are more likely to be set aside unused, or perhaps they will be used differently than intended. As new technologies extend to the bedside and home use, their benefits (both medical and economic) will be lost if they result in incorrect or delayed diagnoses, unexpected office or hospital visits, or more complicated patient treatments. Usability engineering can provide guidance and structure for establishing that the product can be successfully and safely used by the target user in its intended environment. In doing so, it helps companies avoid the unacceptable financial and human costs required to support a suboptimal product, enhances the user experience, and reduces risk by eliminating use errors.

In broad terms, "usability engineering" is the application of human engineering, human factors, and ergonomics to medical devices. Related to "user-centered design," it considers the user and, just as importantly, the environment in which he or she interacts with the device. The goal is to ensure that the product is easy to use (the user can operate it without confusion) and safe to use (the user is unlikely to operate it incorrectly).

Although they all can result in hazards to the user or patient, it is important to differentiate between "use errors," "user errors," "device failures," and "technology-induced errors." "Use errors" are central to usability engineering—an objective term for capturing that an error occurred. Use errors are not insignificant—a review of the U.S. Food and Drug Administration (FDA) medical device incident reports shows that about one-third of the approximately 100,000 incidents reported each year are due to use errors [1]. The terms "user errors" and "device failures" by definition assign blame respectively, to the user or device. Because use error can result from poor product design (e.g., a confusing user interface) the error is not necessarily the user's fault. Device failures, while part of product risk analysis, are addressed through hardware or software engineering and do not depend on the user interaction with the device. "Technology-induced errors" while still use errors, are a newer concept in which the technology itself, or the user's interaction with the technology in a real life setting, results in medical errors [2,3]. Use errors can be categorized as slips, lapses, or mistakes [4]. Some examples of use errors are entering the wrong information (perhaps because a default value was presented and the user did not change it) or disregarding an alarm condition (perhaps because the alarm was not noticed). The abnormal use of a product is not considered a use error. An FDA presentation entitled "The FDA Perspective on Human Factors in Medical Device Software Development" [4] noted some common reasons for use errors:

1. The environment negatively impacts the use of the device (e.g., user is distracted, lighting or noise levels prevent the device from being used as expected).
2. The demands associated with use of the device exceed user's capabilities (i.e., cognitive, physical).
3. The user interface may be contradictory to user's expectation or intuition.
4. The device is used in unexpected ways.
5. The device is used in inappropriate but foreseeable ways, for which adequate controls were not applied.

Repeated use errors will lower confidence in the product and make it less likely to be used as intended. Usability engineering is applied at the earliest phases of product definition and risk management and impacts the design input requirements. These requirements can then be refined and tested throughout the product development process.

7.2 STANDARDS, REFERENCES, AND GUIDANCE RELATED TO USABILITY ENGINEERING

For a device to obtain FDA clearance or a European CE mark, the development process will usually include compliance with IEC 62366 (Medical devices—Application of usability engineering to medical devices) [5]. This international standard defines a method to apply the usability engineering process to medical device design. The usability engineering process is closely tied to risk management, as defined in ISO 14971 (Medical Devices—Application of risk management to medical devices) [6]. Following IEC 62366 should result in an acceptable level of risk according to the approaches described in ISO 14971.

AAMI/ANSI HE75 (Human factors engineering—Design of medical devices) [7] complements the standards and provides a useful reference for the practical application of human factors to design. Its encyclopedic 445 pages cover principles of usability engineering and testing, general advice for good design, and factors to consider during device design.

Because of the large number of reported use errors that lead to a medical incident reports regulatory agencies have increasingly focused their attention on usability engineering. FDA has published usability-related guidance for over a decade (the guidance "Medical Device Use Safety: Incorporating Human Factors in Risk Management" was published in 2000 [8]), and now also has a website dedicated to providing more information on the human factors program [9]. Additionally, FDA has published a draft guidance document "Applying Human Factors and Usability Engineering to Optimize Medical Device Design" [10] that will eventually replace the earlier guidance, describing FDA's approach to human factors and usability engineering in design. While complementing the standards and referencing multiple other FDA guidance documents related to usability, it provides practical information to consider as part of product design and testing. At this time, FDA is reviewing the more than 500 comments received on this draft guidance and incorporating appropriate comments before issuing the final guidance. Although the guidance is not final, it does represent recent thinking on the part of the Agency. A good approach to address the regulations is to be in compliance with IEC 62366 and use the guidance documents and AAMI/ANSI HE75 to develop detailed plans and activities. For regulatory submissions it is always a good idea to provide justification if there are parts of a guidance document with which you do not wish to comply.

7.3 PRACTICAL APPLICATION OF USABILITY ENGINEERING

Usability engineering should be regarded as an iterative process that occurs throughout the product lifecycle, as shown in Figure 7.1. During the product feasibility and planning phases, user research helps determine who the user is and what the product will do for them, and establish the environment in which the product will be used. These research results form the basis of a conceptual design for the product which then is further elaborated in requirements definition. These usability activities are iteratively applied to develop the first set of requirements for product development. For example, after the first cycle of requirement specification, more user research in

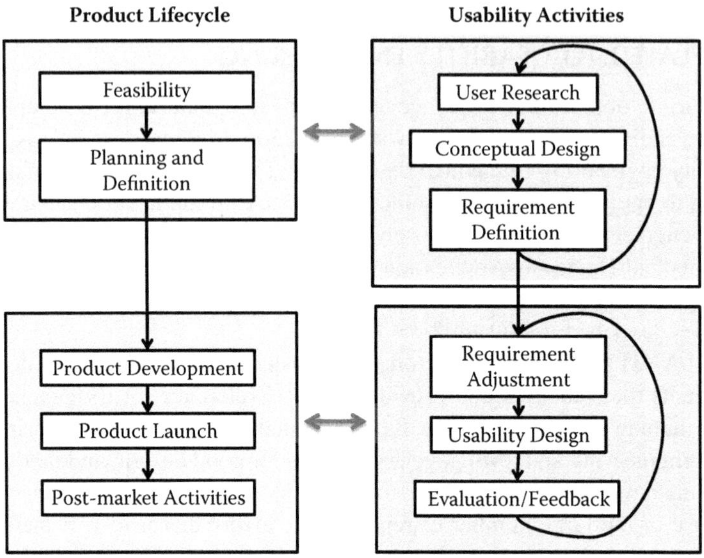

FIGURE 7.1 Links between product lifecycle and usability activities.

the form of a focus group could be applied to the proposed conceptual design/requirements. During the remaining product lifecycle stages, iterative cycles of requirement refinement followed by usability design and evaluation are conducted to continually improve the product, even in the post-market stage. The relationship between design control, usability engineering, and usability evaluations is summarized in Table 7.1.

Usability engineering, as defined in IEC 62366, provides a structured approach to plan, execute, and document the usability activities. The documents produced in compliance with IEC 62366 are listed in Table 7.2. Especially important to the process are the application specification, the consideration of usability risks, the usability specification, and usability evaluation or validation testing.

The usability engineering plan provides an overall approach for usability engineering activities including expected documents, deliverables, and testing strategy. The application specification defines the intended user profile(s), the use environment(s), and patient population(s). The user profiles should consider different educational backgrounds, and physical, demographic, or other attributes that could affect the user's interaction with the product. National or regional differences should be considered as well. This is important not only for device functionality, but for the terminology that is used in the user interface and user materials. The key with user profiles is to differentiate user types that are expected to have different approaches to or interactions with the device. Because of these variations, each user profile identified will be tested in the later usability evaluations. In the medical setting, some distinct user profiles may be: physicians, nurses, technicians, and patients, because each of these users will approach a product with a different level of understanding and have different contexts for product use. In a home use setting, a pediatric patient may have a different user profile than his or her caregiver or parent. There is no substitute for direct discussions with users to understand, even before a prototype device exists,

TABLE 7.1
How Design Control Phases Link to Usability

Design Control	Usability Engineering	Usability Evaluations
Feasibility/Concept		
• User research • Conceptual design	• User research on user profiles, environments, competitive products • Documentation of usability evaluations	• Cognitive walkthrough • Competitive comparison • Interviews • Focus groups
Development Planning		
	• Usability engineering plan	• Usability evaluation strategy
Design Inputs		
• Criteria and requirements • Risk analyses • Usability specifications	• Application specification • Use risk analyses • Usability specification • Usability objectives • Documentation of usability evaluations	• Cognitive walkthrough • Interviews • Focus groups
Design Outputs		
	• Usability design • Mock-ups • Prototypes • Simulations • Documentation of usability evaluations	• Cognitive walkthrough • Formative assessment tests
Design Verification and Validation		
	• Usability specification Verification report • Usability validation report	• Usability specification verification • Usability validation
Design Transfer to Production		
	• Usability engineering file	
Design Changes		
	• Usability engineering file	• Post-market studies • Customer feedback

the types of products or technologies they currently use, and further, to explore what they like and do not like about them. The information gathered in these discussions will have an impact later on user materials and training.

Use environments, such as lighting conditions, space requirements, and noise levels must also be considered. For example, think about if the product would be used in a high workload (stressed) or relaxed setting, if the patient is moving or bedridden, if the lighting will be bright or low or both. Will other devices be used concurrently with the product? Finally, consider if the product might migrate to a different use environment. Keep in mind that, as with the user profiles, use environments may vary regionally and this will have an impact on the usability evaluations.

TABLE 7.2
Contents of the Usability Engineering File

Usability engineering plan
Application specification
Risk assessment
Usability specification
Usability validation plan or protocol
Usability validation report

Note: The documents produced in the usability engineering process are compiled into a usability engineering file. These include not only the specific usability document prescribed by IEC 62366 but the related risk documentation.

The application specification must also describe the patient population upon which the device will be used. What are the limitations of these patients? For example, is the device intended to be used on frail patients who have mobility challenges? These factors tie into the risk management process.

There is a close connection between the usability engineering and risk management processes. After the application specification has been generated, use-related errors can be systematically identified. First, gather known hazards (e.g., complaints) about similar products. FDA databases (Manufacturer and User Facility Device Experience or MAUDE [11], Medical Device Report [12], and the Medical Product Safety Network or MedSun [13]) list adverse events filed for products registered in the United States. These are grouped by product code, so it may be necessary to search the FDA product classification database first for the appropriate product code(s). Then search the FDA adverse event and recall databases for reported adverse events and recalls.

The risk management process provides a structure for thoroughly identifying hazards related to the product, then defining means to mitigate or control the related risks. The usability engineering process focuses specifically on use-related risks, identifying anticipated and unanticipated use-related hazards. These types of hazards are distinct from hazards that arise from the device itself (e.g., electromagnetic interference, biocompatibility, sterility). Use-related hazards that are identified during the normal top-down risk assessment and failure mode and effects analyses (FMEAs) should be identified as such for consideration in the usability specification.

The application specification and risk assessments are used to create design input requirements that are captured in the product and software requirements specifications. IEC 62366 also calls out a usability specification. The usability specification should identify the desired use scenarios and also describe the worst-case use scenarios—conditions under which the user is more likely, because of pressure, confusion, etc. to make a mistake. These will be useful for determining usability evaluation conditions later. The usability specification also identifies "primary operating functions"—defined as either frequently used functions or functions that are related to safety. The specific requirements related to these functions are then described so that they can be implemented. Often these primary operating functions are the focus of usability assessment studies and study participants will be asked to perform tasks related to these functions to demonstrate that the risks related to them have been mitigated.

A usability study should be treated like any other formal study, with an approved plan or protocol and carefully designed test forms for collecting data. The results of the testing are described in a usability validation report. All documentation related to usability (shown in Table 7.2) is compiled into the usability engineering file. Similarly, risk assessments, specifications, and verification results generated in the usability engineering process are referenced in the risk management file. Ultimately, the safe and effective use of the final device design, and a demonstration that the risks have been mitigated to an acceptable level, is confirmed in a usability validation study.

7.4 USABILITY EVALUATIONS

Usability evaluations explore and confirm that the profiled users can operate the device as expected when used in scenarios and environments that are as close to realistic as possible. Usability evaluations should be conducted iteratively throughout the life of the product along with use-based risk analysis. As with user discussions, it is best to start evaluations as early as possible in the development process. Table 7.1 shows the relationship of usability evaluations to design controls throughout the development process.

Early, defined as "formative," testing can help to avoid delays and complications later in development, when the product is at a mature stage and more difficult to redesign. Formative testing may use early simulations of the product (or a competitive or similar product), involve five to eight users, and will not have acceptance criteria. The goals of formative testing are to elicit user feedback, identify unexpected use errors, identify new risks, and provide insights into how to improve the product. Also, formative usability test results can serve as a benchmark for subsequent usability testing. Table 7.3 summarizes types of formative testing that can be used during product development.

TABLE 7.3
Types of Formative Usability Testing

Testing Type	Description
Exploratory testing/ cognitive walkthrough	Explore concepts using mock-ups of the user interface such as drawings, computer wireframes, or foam models. Walk through proposed functionality and workflows with the user and solicit feedback regarding difficulties they notice in using the device.
Comparison (contrast) testing	Have the user indicate their preferences to two or more design alternatives—such as button size/location or icons.
Competitive testing	Test and gather feedback using a competitive product.
Assessment testing	Ask users to perform particular tasks using simulations or early prototypes. For example, do they notice the audible alerts and act accordingly? Additionally some tasks may focus on the ability of users to acquire needed information from the user manual (e.g., how to interpret an error code and fix the problem).

Source: Human Factors Engineering—Design of Medical Devices. *ANSI/AAMI Standard, HE75*, 2009. With permission.

Summative usability tests are more formal than formative tests and typically are performed as part of the final product validation. The AAMI/ANSI HE75 term *summative usability* test is synonymous with FDA's term *usability validation* test. Such testing should be conducted on production or pilot-production units and should include any user manuals, product training materials, and/or direct user training that are anticipated for commercial use. The testing will evaluate the clarity of the information presented to the user. If no or minimal training is envisioned, then usability testing will confirm this approach is viable. Usability evaluations have a different focus and goal than clinical validation studies. Clinical validation demonstrates the clinical performance of the device, while usability must capture use by the different user profiles. Because of this, the two studies are not typically combined.

7.5 USABILITY VALIDATION TESTING STEPS

7.5.1 Setting Usability Objectives

Usability validation testing helps to provide evidence that the device meets user needs. Carefully planning ahead of the testing should consider and establish clear, testable usability objectives (also known as *usability goals* or *usability requirements*). For example, instead of saying the "calibration is easy for the user to perform," a requirement could be "90% of intended users can successfully complete the calibration step on their first attempt." Usability objectives should be related to the primary operating functions (frequently used functions and the functions related to safety). Some common elements of usability goals include:

- Success rates for completing assigned tasks
- Time to complete tasks
- Number of times user needs to refer to user manual
- Correct interpretation of information (e.g., ability to find and interpret troubleshooting guide in user manual)
- User ratings (e.g., Likert scale or other comparative ratings).

These objectives will be evaluated in the study protocol.

7.5.2 Planning and Protocols

Similar to other studies and as required in IEC 62366, usability validations should have a study plan/protocol. AAMI/ANSI HE75 [7] recommends the following protocol sections:

1. Purpose
2. Setting
3. Participants
4. Description of test unit (e.g., prototypes or simulations)
5. Methodology or test protocol
6. Task

7. Usability objectives
8. Data collection
9. Data analysis
10. Reporting

The protocol should consider if an actual or simulated setting will be used. It should provide a detailed justification for why a simulated environment is adequate. How many different user groups and how many participants per group will be tested? The different user groups should have been identified earlier in the usability engineering process (in the application specification). The number of participants needed for usability studies depends upon the purpose of the study, the number of user profile types, and the expected rates of use errors. AAMI/ANSI HE75 [7] provides an Annex for testing sample size statistical justification. Generally, testing should include at least 15 participants from each user profile type. A study with 15 participants is estimated to detect a minimum of 90% of the problems that might exist in a software product [14], which may be why the FDA draft guidance document recommends including at least 15 participants of each user profile type. AAMI/ANSI HE75 [7] recommends at least 15–20 participants per distinct user profile group in the summative usability validation study, but points out that other human factors professionals advocate larger sample sizes (30–100) to detect a higher percentage of usability defects and to provide higher statistical power. As summative usability testing is typically provided as part of the regulatory submissions, the sample sizes chosen must be justified in the final usability validation report. It is also important to note that the testing participants should closely simulate or fit the appropriate user profile. The draft FDA guidance [10] specifically states that employees should not be test participants, as their knowledge about the product will influence how they use it (the exception being the rare cases where all users necessarily are employees of the manufacturer).

Another critical aspect of the usability validation test is the selection of tasks that the participants will be asked to do. This should be based upon the usability objectives and the risk analyses. It is especially important to show that functions related to device safety can meet the usability objectives. It may be desirable to have failures built in to the protocol to see if the user can identify and recover from them. For example, purposefully provide the device with low batteries to see if the participant ignores or reacts to the associated warnings and alarms. Some other examples include asking the participant to: calibrate the device, work through the user interface to enter information, read the results and document what they believe the result means, and troubleshoot a device error.

In addition to the subjective data (e.g., exit interview feedback), the testing should collect objective performance data, such as the number of attempts needed to accomplish a task or the time taken to complete a task. The protocol should describe how use failures are defined and recorded (for example, if a user is allowed three tries to complete a task before categorizing their effort as a use failure).

How the data is collected is critical for minimizing bias. Often an objective third party, known as an *unobtrusive observer*, will watch (but not interfere with) the testing. The observer may also make time measurements as tasks are completed. While using an observer is important for data collection, it can also be a source of bias. To reduce test bias, AAMI/ANSI HE75 [7] recommends that observers:

1. Do not lead, prompt, or help participants in performing the assigned tasks.
2. Make only neutral comments; do not speculate on what the user is thinking. Try not to engage in conversations with the participant.
3. Reply to participants who ask "Can I do that?" with "What do you think would happen if you did that?" or "Please consult the user manual."
4. Be aware of body language and facial expressions when interacting with the participant.
5. Talk only as needed to clarify and run the evaluation; try not to interrupt the participant.
6. End the task if the participant is lost. Criteria should be defined in the protocol (e.g., no more than three attempts or no more than 5 minutes) for ending tasks.

7.5.3 Study Execution

Once the usability validation protocol has been approved, the study coordinator should consider the logistics of how to successfully complete the study. Investigational Review Board (IRB) approval will likely be required if the investigational device is going to be used on actual patients. However, if the usability study only focuses on the user interface and no diagnosis or treatment is made, IRB review is usually not required. Other study logistics are similar to those required for a clinical study: recruiting participants, identifying testing locations, planning for a session, and designing data capture forms. However, the desire to objectively capture the user's experience may lead to additional potential activities such as including an unobtrusive observer or video recording the session. Other elements may include planned failure or alarm incidents to observe the user's interactions in worst-case scenarios and an exit interview and/or survey for the participants. Throughout the study appropriate data collection and good documentation practices should be followed to ensure data integrity.

AAMI/ANSI HE75 [7] notes the following common usability study errors that should be reviewed with the testing staff prior to study execution:

1. Not pretesting the protocol (pretesting or conducting a "dry run" can help remove ambiguous task statements and instructions and can help ensure that the test runs smoothly)
2. Leading or biasing participants
3. Helping participants complete the tasks
4. Talking too much or not watching carefully
5. Rushing participants
6. Making participants feel inferior
7. Not making sessions friendly and interactive, and
8. Not keeping track of timing and having to rush to finish all tasks in the protocol.

The first step in conducting a usability evaluation is usually providing information to the participant about the study and obtaining their informed consent (normally this will also include a non-disclosure clause). In some cases a pre-study questionnaire collects the participant's demographic or other data. Then the participant will be given the same training as expected in commercial use (for example, the participant is asked to read the user manual). Keep in mind that it may be necessary to adapt training to different user profiles and environments and that the evaluations may highlight these issues. Once ready, the participant will be observed as they proceed through the series of planned tasks. Seeing users make mistakes is extremely valuable insight into the product usability. It not only illuminates design or workflow problems, but provides an opportunity to see how the user might try to recover from an error or unexpected interaction. At the end of the testing it may be helpful to conduct an exit interview and/or give the user a questionnaire asking for their feedback on the product. FDA's guidance has indicated that user studies may include subjective feedback from the test to establish if, for example, the users understood how and when they had made errors, and if the instructions provided helped them to realize the error. This can provide insights into the user's interpretation of the experience versus their observed behavior. Often, a user survey is also conducted. Any user surveys should have acceptance criteria (an expected average score, for example) defined in the protocol.

7.5.4 Data Analysis and Reporting

Usability validation data analysis typically involves descriptive statistics (e.g., the mean time to complete a task or percent of subjects that completed a task on the first try). Interpretation of the summative usability test results should include both the subjective and the objective data. In addition to verifying usability objectives, an analysis and discussion of any problems identified, "close calls," and use failures should be made in the usability validation report. The draft FDA guidance [10] provides more information regarding interpretation of results as well as an outline of a Human Factors/Usability Engineering Report.

The usability evaluations reports should be included in the Usability Engineering File. These reports will be reviewed during inspections by FDA and notified bodies. Additionally some of these reports may be included in the application to FDA for clearance or approval of the medical device.

7.6 CONCLUSION

There is an increasing focus on usability in product development and case studies report on its practical implementation [15]. Professional societies, especially in the area of health informatics, are recognizing the need to consider human factors, forming working groups to study and improve usability [16]. Usability engineering is an iterative and on-going process which, due to the variability in user profiles and use environments, is especially important for mobile point-of-care devices. Thinking through the users, their environment, the mistakes they may make, and then repeatedly testing the updated product designs with the defined user profiles can ensure that the final point-of-care product will be accepted and used as intended. The usability and risk management processes provide a structure for ensuring these evaluations are documented and thorough. There are also numerous standards and guidance documents that will help a company to formulate their formative and summative usability evaluations. The growing awareness of usability engineering and the need to understand and mitigate use errors will help ensure health monitoring and diagnostic technologies are successfully extended to the point of care and to the patients themselves.

REFERENCES

1. Patterson P.A. and North R.A. Fitting Human Factors in the Product Development Process. *Medical Device & Diagnostic Industry,* http://www.mddionline.com/article/fitting-human-factors-product-development-process [accessed 15 September 2013].
2. Koppel, R., J.P. Metlay, A. Cohen, B. Abaluck, R. Localio, S.E. Kimmel, and B.L. Strom. 2005. Role of Computerized Physician Order Entry Systems in Facilitating Medication Errors. *JAMA* 293:1197–03.
3. Ammenwerth, E. and N.T. Shaw. 2004. Bad Informatics Can Kill—Is Evaluation the Answer? *Methods of Information Medicine* 44(1):1–3.
4. FDA. *The FDA Perspective on Human Factors in Medical Device Software Development,* 1 February, 2012, http://www.fda.gov/downloads/medicaldevices/deviceregulationandguidance/humanfactors/ucm290561.pdf [accessed 16 September 2013].
5. Medical Devices—Application of Usability Engineering to Medical Devices. *IEC Standard 62366*, 2007.
6. Medical devices—Application of risk management to medical devices. *ISO Standard* 14971, 2012.
7. Human Factors Engineering—Design of Medical Devices. *ANSI/AAMI Standard, HE75*, 2009.
8. FDA document UM094461. *Medical Device Safety: Incorporating Human Factors Engineering into Risk Management,* http://www.fda.gov/downloads/MedicalDevices/.../ucm094461.pdf [accessed 15 September 2013].
9. FDA Human factors website, http://www.fda.gov/MedicalDevices/DeviceRegulationandGuidance/HumanFactors/default.htm [accessed 13 September, 2013].
10. FDA document UCM259748. *Applying Human Factors and Usability Engineering to OptimizeMedicalDeviceDesign,* http://www.fda.gov/MedicalDevices/DeviceRegulationandGuidance/GuidanceDocuments/ucm259748.htm [accessed 13 September, 2013].
11. FDA. MAUDE—Manufacturer and User Facility Device Experience Database, http://www.accessdata.fda.gov/scripts/cdrh/cfdocs/cfMAUDE/search.CFM [accessed 16 September 2013].
12. FDA. Medical Device Reporting Database, http://www.accessdata.fda.gov/scripts/cdrh/cfdocs/cfmdr/search.CFM [accessed 16 September 2013].
13. FDA. MedSun: Medical Product Safety Network, http://www.fda.gov/MedicalDevices/Safety/MedSunMedicalProductSafetyNetwork/ucm127686.htm [accessed 16 September 2013].
14. Faulkner, L. 2003. Beyond the Five-User Assumption: Benefits of Increased Sample Sizes in Usability Testing. *Behavior Research Methods, Instruments, and Computers* 35(3):379–383.
15. van der Peijl J., Klein J., Grass C., and Freudenthal A. 2012. Design for Risk Control: The Role of Usability Engineering in the Management of Use-Related Risks. *J. Biomed. Inform* August 45(4):795–812.

16. International Medical Informatics Association. Human Factors Engineering for Healthcare Informatics. *International Medical Informatics Association*, http://www.imia-medinfo.org/new2/node/142 [accessed 19 September 2013].

8 Translating Sensor Technology into the Medical Device Environment

Robert D. Black

CONTENTS

8.1 INTRODUCTION

The translation of a sensor technology into clinical medicine is a complex and multifaceted undertaking [1–4]. In addition to challenges in the discovery phase, there are regulatory, reimbursement, and physician acceptance hurdles to clear. The latter challenges are often not considered in research-oriented journal articles and authors of such articles run the risk of reporting on developments that may ultimately be sterile in a translational sense. As research funding sources become increasingly challenging to obtain, work that purports to support new capabilities in human medicine must be complete in the sense of being able to clear all hurdles that will be arrayed against it. This is not to say that there is not a vital role for pure research projects, but work that is "justified" by an implied payback in advancing human health must evolve with a full recognition and acceptance of what that entails. Some questions that should be asked, even at the earliest stages of development are:

- Will the product fit into existing reimbursement codes?
- Will the product be approved by the FDA when a tractable clinical trial is completed?
- If the device is an implantable sensor, how is it implanted and can it be included with an existing procedure?
- Does the device fit with existing medical training and practices and if not what is the learning curve for acceptance?
- If the device involves sensor data, specifically, how will that data be used to influence patient care?
- Can the device be manufactured in a cost-effective way?
- Does the implanted device meet the "burden of inconvenience" test, meaning that the information provided is unique and valuable and cannot be obtained by less invasive means (e.g., a blood test)?

Starting with a review of some of the essential considerations involved in the regulatory process, several examples of sensor-based technologies that are now in wide use with patients will be noted. Finally, some future trends that rely on sensor-based devices, as projected by the FDA, will be mentioned. In the end, this article will have succeeded if it provides the reader with a better appreciation of the multifaceted environment in which discoveries that seek to be translated into human medicine must navigate.

8.2 THE FDA PROCESS FOR MEDICAL DEVICES

In the United States, the Food and Drug Administration (FDA) oversees commercialization of medical devices [5]. In Europe, for example, the Medical Device Directive (MDD) leads to harmonization of standards, but each country applies the MDD for consistency with national goals. Therefore, generalizing, the regulations surrounding the commercialization of devices is a nation-by-nation process and herein we will focus on the particular requirements of the FDA. The rules established for the FDA are based on laws contained in the Code of Federal Regulations (CFR).

How the device is to be used: When speaking of regulatory control of medical devices one must first define both the intended use and indication for use. Though similar, the concepts differ and the latter is in some sense a subset of the former. Intended use refers to the overall goal in using the device and can be fairly generic (21 CFR 801.4). The indication(s) for use (e.g., 21 CFR 814.20(b)(3)(i)) refer to: "A general description of the disease or condition the device will diagnose, treat, prevent, cure, or mitigate, including a description of the patient population for which the device is intended." Therefore a given device can in principle have many indications for use and each new use must be evaluated in terms of whether it creates new questions of safety and efficacy and, if so, the device maker will need to provide data establishing safety and efficacy (possibly clinical data). Developers of medical sensors, therefore, must navigate this preliminary classification question and delineate clearly the role of the sensor and how it will affect patient health.

8.2.1 Safety and Efficacy

The essence of what the FDA regulates is the safety of the device: does it have potential to harm the patient directly or through information it provides that affects patient care, and does the device accomplish its indication for use. A common misconception is that a product that "doesn't touch the patient" is not a medical device. But even software that records patient medical records, for example, is subject to regulation (clearly if the information provided by the software is faulty, that could affect patient care and well-being). Even if a sensor system does not perform a direct diagnostic or therapeutic function it may still be classified as a medical device if, again, it has the potential to alter patient care. An element of a telemetry system, were it to malfunction, could provide erroneous data to a physician and lead to improper interventions being taken with a patient. Sensors in medical devices must have rigorous calibration records demonstrating the accuracy of the sensor for the intended use for the duration of a diagnostic or therapeutic procedure. If, during development, a sensor designed for a medical application is not deemed to be accurate enough then a secondary method of calibration would have to be established. For example, continuous glucose monitors rely on calibration by established glucometers.

8.2.2 Establishing a Predicate

Although most new medical devices have novel features, it is often the case that they share an indication for use with an established commercial device: a predicate device. Identifying a predicate device provides a distinct advantage when pursuing device commercialization since the burden of proof is lessened. In effect, one can take advantage of an existing track record of safety and efficacy. But how close must such a predicate be? There is no clear-cut means of making such a determination and the device maker must consult with the FDA so as to work out a development plan that will be accepted when the device is proffered for regulatory scrutiny. This is the most challenging concept for inventors and researchers seeking to introduce sensors into the medical environment. Whereas novelty is essential for the process of invention and seeking patent protection, it works against the concept of predicate-use scenarios. Researchers are rewarded for devising new and different sensors that can, in theory, be useful in advancing medicine. Too often the promise, sometimes hype, is not commensurate with the likelihood of translation into medical practice. False hope and optimism can be generated when the stakeholders in an invention have not paid adequate attention to the entire chain of events that must be addressed when moving from the lab to the clinic. One often sees cautionary comments, indicating that many years separate a discovery from implementation in the clinic, but interested parties are left wondering, "if not now, when?" Premature announcements of potential medical significance, frankly, serve no purpose and should be eschewed.

An important caveat when speaking of predicate devices is to establish the risk classification of the predicate. There are two overlapping risk assessment categories, the first being whether the device is significant or non-significant risk (SR or NSR). Here risk covers both risk to the patient and the operator of the device. Additionally, devices are categorized into three classes. Class I devices are products that are not for a substantive use in preventing impairment of human health and that do not present a potentially unreasonable risk of patient injury. Examination gloves are Class I devices. Class II devices include higher technology products that do not by themselves maintain life, but nonetheless can have an important impact on patient care. MRI machines are Class II devices. Class III devices are used in supporting or sustaining human life or are substantially important in preventing impairment of human health. Novel implants such as neurostimulators are in this category. Obviously Class III devices are SR. Class II devices can be SR or NSR. Class I devices are NSR.

8.2.3 Regulatory Pathway

Focusing on medical sensors, there are two primary potential procedural pathways for gaining regulatory certification. The first is commonly called a *510(k)* and the second a *PMA* (premarket approval). Devices are "cleared" in the 510(k) pathway and "approved" via the PMA pathway. There is a third pathway, referred to as *de novo* that can serve as an intermediate route as discussed below. Understanding how to navigate the approval pathway is a primary undertaking in the translational process. A 510(k) device is one that has a demonstrable predicate, is Class I or II, and may be SR or NSR. If a device is determined to be SR, then a formal application, termed an *Investigational Device Exemption* (IDE), must be submitted to the FDA before clinical data is acquired in support of a device application. In the IDE the sponsor lays out the reasoning behind a proposed clinical investigation, summarizes laboratory or animal data, etc. The aim is to explain to the FDA how the proposed approach will answer questions germane to the clearance process. Until the IDE is approved, no human research is permitted. If a device is NSR, approval for clinical work may be obtained through an Institutional Review Board, which exist within many hospitals and may also be separate, private organizations. Determining *whether* a sensor-based device clearance requires human test data is another important consideration when evaluating clinical potential.

Frequently a medical sensor would be expected to fall into the 510(k) category, but what about a sensor type that truly is novel as applied to medical science? What about a sensor device that has the attributes of a Class II device, is NSR, and yet has no direct predicate in the market? With only two pathways available, 510(k) and PMA, such a device would have to be regulated through the PMA route and be Class III, even though it may be extremely safe and effective. In an effort to resolve this logical impasse the *de novo* pathway was initiated by the FDA. A *de novo* device is one that is viewed to be low risk and yet does not have an indication for use that matches currently marketed products. Effectively, the device becomes its own predicate... *de novo*. The process of obtaining *de novo* approval is comparable to that for a 510(k) device, but the FDA may invoke an advisory panel review, which adds time to the process.

Devices that are both high risk and non-substantially equivalent to a predicate device will be regulated via the PMA pathway. A PMA application requires compilation and presentation of considerable amounts of information. This includes a complete description of the device and components, photos and engineering diagrams, a detailed description of the methods, facilities, and controls used to manufacture the device, the proposed labeling and advertising literature, training materials, software documentation, biocompatibility information, and references to applicable standards. A summary of all clinical, animal, and bench data is also required. An advisory panel is often assembled to provide an external review of the device and an inspection of manufacturing facilities will be arranged. Finally, after PMA approval the FDA maintains market surveillance rights as the product is commercialized. The PMA process can take years and cost millions or tens-of-millions of dollars. This is a substantial hurdle for novel, untried technology, such as a new sensor system, to clear and the process focuses attention on the market potential of the device.

8.2.4 Independent Device Testing

Since any new medical device raises questions of safety, it is essential to have independent bodies test and verify compliance with safety standards. For example, with respect to biocompatibility a device may need to undergo toxicology, sensitization, and irritation testing if it is to be implanted or even just contact the skin. There are several laboratories that perform these testing services. For a medical sensor that must operate in a biological environment, additional testing of its functional state during exposure to that environment must be included. Devices must also adhere to a set of technical standards set forth in IEC 60601 (International Electrotechnical Commission) and the device maker must show empirical evidence that the device has passed the safety and functional tests set forth in this standard. The so-called third edition rules under this standard outline significant new rules for home-use devices. Thus medical sensors in home use products face additional testing in order to demonstrate compliance. The time and cost involved in biocompatibility and IEC testing can also be significant.

8.2.5 Some Specific Examples of Sensor Characteristics That Evoke Regulatory Decision Points

1. Implanted sensor breakage or migration: There is strong interest in diagnostic sensors that can reside in or near bodily organs and provide feedback on medical conditions (e.g., blood pressure in the heart or serum glucose levels in diabetics). In addition to the question of how to place such sensors, that is the surgical approach, the issues of how to keep such sensors in the desired location and avoid damage to the sensor that could expose the patient to risk must be addressed. Typically sensors will have some means of retention associated with the outer package. This could take the form of a feature that allows for suturing or some sort of adhesive coating that works against sensor slippage. If the sensor is near the skin surface, will it be subjected to forces that could potentially fracture the device? If the sensor does move away from the point of placement, might it inflict damage on nearby tissues or organs? For instance a sensor that resides in the heart or nearby large vessels must be evaluated for its potential to create an

embolism should it come free. If the sensor components include potentially toxic components, testing should account for the possibility of breakage and leakage in the patient.

2. Biocompatibility: In addition to the physical concerns stated above for implanted sensors, biological compatibility must also be established. The general requirements are summarized in the ISO-10993 standards. For implanted devices cytotoxicity (toxic effects on cells), irritation, and sensitization are routinely studied. Additionally, based on the component materials questions about carcinogenicity and genotoxicity may arise. These latter tests can extend the time horizon for biocompatibility testing in general and should be factored into the timeline of the translational plan. The use of novel materials that have not been utilized in already-marketed medical devices can be particularly challenging since regulatory agencies are unable to derive guidance from previous studies in gauging new risks that novel materials may present. Extensive *in vitro* and animal testing will be expected for new implantable substances.
3. Biofouling: Separate from the effects of an implanted sensor on the body are the effects residing on the body may have on the sensor. For implanted medical sensors, key to the success is the need to ensure reliable performance when exposed to living tissue and fluids. The term *biofouling* has gained common usage as a description of the buildup of proteins and fibroblasts that accompany the body's immune reaction against foreign objects. Effectively, the body attempts to wall off the foreign material and the growth layer is typically 100 microns thick or more. This layer is problematic for any device that seeks to sample serum or blood, for example, since it acts as a diffusion barrier. Implanted glucose sensors provide a case in point.
4. Electromagnetic interference: Electronically active medical devices must work in the expected range of environments to which they will be exposed and also not interfere with other electronic systems in the health care setting. The rules differ based on whether the device is intended for home use or hospital use. Both IEC (e.g., IEC 60601-1-2) and FCC requirements must be met. Typically testing by a third party is required to demonstrate that a medical device complies with existing industry and local regulations. With the ubiquity of wireless communication devices operating in the ~2.4 GHz band, sensor systems that rely on wireless connections must avoid packet collisions that could corrupt data flow. The Wireless Medical Telemetry Service was established by the FCC in an attempt to provide a less crowded frequency space for medical devices, but the advantages of accessing the wide array of existing commercial products operating in the WiFi and Bluetooth bands means that the issue has not gone away.
5. Telemetry: The growth of sensors systems for portable monitoring has prompted the FDA to issue new guidance (e.g., Wireless Medical Telemetry Risks and Recommendations). In addition to the EMI concerns noted above, the security of patient data is a significant area of regulatory scrutiny. The Health Insurance Portability and Accountability Act (HIPPA) includes a set of directives that put strict limits on the sharing of patient data. In this

context, even the initials of the patient, for instance, cannot be transferred in transmissions that may be subject to unintended viewing by unauthorized persons. Uninformed device developers have encountered significant hurdles when attempting to commercialize "apps" that cross the boundary into the definition of a medical device because the app collects and transmits sensitive patient data.

6. Clinical utility: Strictly speaking, the FDA evaluates medical devices for safety and efficacy. Does the device perform as stated and is it safe for the intended use? A separate question is whether the device performs a necessary or useful medical function. This is a question faced often by medical sensor technology and although the FDA does not formally comment on "commercial potential," it is common to have a requirement that the device must demonstrate utility, most commonly as the result of a well-run clinical study. Just as with drug studies, devices must show superior performance to a placebo in order to gain regulatory clearance. Additionally, even if the device performs a useful function, is there an existing, easier means for obtaining the same information? A good rule of thumb for implanted sensors, for instance, is that if you can acquire the same data by taking a blood sample, the implanted sensor will not gain traction. Even in cases such as the development around implanted glucose sensors, thus far the older and accepted glucometers that rely on a blood draw retain a controlling role in the management of diabetic patients. Clinical utility is perhaps the single most underanalyzed aspect of the translational process.

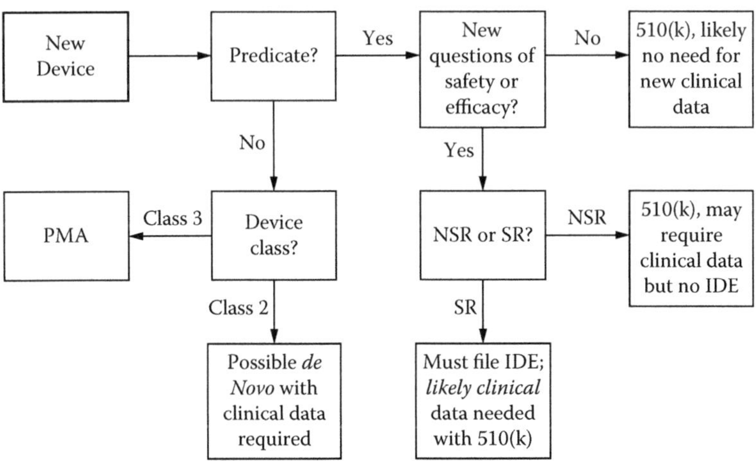

FIGURE 8.1 Representative flowchart for assessing likely disposition of a new medical device. (*Note*: This diagram should not be viewed as being absolute and the device sponsor should consult with the FDA in order to ascertain the appropriate procedural pathway.)

What follows is a short list of case examples demonstrating FDA pathway, design considerations, and the process of translation in general.

Glucose Sensing

There are roughly 800,000 type 1 diabetics in the United States and a portion of the estimated 26 million type 2 diabetics who require regular insulin infusions. Insulin, working with serotonin, enables cells to transport glucose through the cell membrane to meet metabolic demand. An insulin injection provides a bolus to the patient and this is sub-optimal in terms of proper serum glucose maintenance. There are current developments aimed at alternative means for introducing insulin, such as inhalers, but the outcome is the same: a large pulse of insulin, which is not how the body can best utilize it. The development of implanted insulin pumps was viewed as a significant advance, as they enable effectively "on demand" supplies of insulin, providing a more natural delivery means. Missing still is a means for feedback that adjusts insulin release based on serum glucose levels. Ergo the vigorous pursuit of an implantable glucose sensor (IGS) that would allow for a closed-loop system with feedback: a true artificial pancreas using only electronic devices.

Most IGS devices that have been proposed envision relatively simple placements under the skin. Yet ultimate removal of and longevity of the sensor are obvious concerns. In terms of "fit" within existing medical practice, an IGS would find fairly ready acceptance. Still, the change in diabetic management that such a device would imply is not to be underestimated. The question of cost-effective manufacturing depends almost entirely on the longevity of the device within the body. Finally, the "burden of inconvenience" test in the case of an IGS would initially seem to be clear-cut. A device that frees a patient from multiple daily blood draws and enables consistent and automated insulin management would be a true advance indeed. But as the various challenges above that face a successful IGS are weighed in comparison with cheap, accurate, and reliable modern glucometers (a "simple blood test"), it is easier to understand why it does not yet exist in medical practice.

What about FDA regulation of an IGS? There is little question that such devices would face a PMA pathway once sufficient clinical data could be collected. The complexity of the software needed to enable automated means for controlling an insulin pump would draw substantial scrutiny. The inherent risk involved in controlling insulin levels is so high, that the device manufacturer will face a very rigorous clinical trial and approval process. And the FDA reserves the right to perform post-market surveillance on PMA devices as a means for checking on the device's performance in the field. It is unlikely that any manufacturer, even a large public company, would undertake that level of burden lightly. To highlight the challenge involved, current so-called continuous glucose monitors (CGM), which are percutaneous sensors that stay in place for 3–7 days, must be independently calibrated using conventional glucometers and the FDA does not allow them to be used without such calibration. An IGS that still requires frequent calibration with a conventional glucometer would be underwhelming, to say the least, and thus the challenge of FDA approval is significant for these devices.

CGM has dominated the recent literature. Though not strictly based on implantable sensors, in the sense of a true IGS, these devices have nonetheless established themselves as "the best alternative" in pursuit of the goal of continuous feedback to an insulin pump for adaptive insulin regulation. Several clinical trials [6–10] have established the utility of this approach and the FDA has cleared devices for this purpose. Investigators have started to examine the additional potential benefits of tighter glucose control for patients with co-morbid disease. Hermanides et al. [11] used CGM in a study of hyperglycemic myocardial infarction patients, concluding that: "Although a promising tool for in-hospital hyperglycemia therapy, (CGM) needs improvement before continuing to large-scale randomized controlled trials." Klupa et al. [12] evaluated the apparent benefit of CGM for cystic fibrosis patients. Development on new formats for percutaneous glucose sensors continues (e.g., [13–17]).

There is little doubt that CGM enabled by percutaneous sensors has gained ground and produced real benefits for many diabetics. Gough et al. [18] point out that none of these devices has been cleared by the FDA as a primary standard and they must still be calibrated using conventional glucometers. Using a porcine model, Gough et al. implanted devices using glucose oxidase chemistry and found: "(i) acceptable long-term biocompatibility, assessed after 18-month implant periods; (ii) immobilized enzyme life exceeding 1 year; (iii) battery life exceeding 1 year; (iv) electronic circuitry reliability and telemetry performance; (v) sensor mechanical robustness including long-term maintenance of hermeticity; (vi) stability of the electrochemical detector structure; and (vii) acceptability and tolerance of the animals to the implanted device." This study may be viewed as a proof-of-concept demonstration that the salient technical challenges facing fully implantable glucose sensors can be met. In addition to amperometric approaches, the use of fluorescent reporters has been explored with some success in laboratory and animal studies [19–26], but translational work is not as advanced.

Capsule Endoscopy

Capsule endoscopy is the term applied to a device with a miniature camera that can be swallowed, allowing for filming inside the GI tract. Though not an implantable sensor, most of the same concerns about biocompatibility, hermeticity, and data collection obtain. The leader in this field is Given Imaging (now a division of Covidien), an entity that successfully traversed the route from small startup to public company. The device, called *Pill Cam*, has been in common use for many years and thus no discrete listing of clinical studies using it is tractable (a Pubmed search on capsule endoscopy will be rewarding to the reader). The Pill Cam device makes use of a CCD camera and LED light sources. The medical need it addressed initially was to provide physicians with a view of the small intestine, which could not be accessed directly by endoscopic means. The device sends images taken at a preset frequency to a recorder worn by the patient during the transit time of the capsule through his or her body. The physician is then able to review these images in a movie-loop format with some location/position data in addition to anatomical landmark identification. Pill Cam received 510(k) clearance with a relatively small human clinical trial. There is no question that the short duration of time in the body as well as the ability to encase the entire device in a biocompatible plastic simplified this process. An interesting question is whether the device would be viewed as substantially equivalent today, as it was a decade ago. At very least it is an interesting case study of the interplay of risk, efficacy, and predicate weighting. Reimbursement for capsule endoscopy was not immediately forthcoming, however medical demand blossomed and physician adoption forcefully pushed aside any question that the device would be broadly covered. This product had to, essentially, define a new subfield of gastroenterology and it had to gain favor with GI professional societies. But it started with a product that is comparably easy to manufacture and deploy and thus serves as a useful case study for those interested in translational medical devices development.

Cochlear Implant

The cochlear implant is a sensor-based technology that evolved over decades and it was eventually approved as a PMA device. It is an interesting example of how sometimes ideas must wait for technical evolution before becoming practical in medicine. Wilson et al. [27] provided an excellent history of the development of the cochlear implant, which the authors rightly called *the most successful current neural prosthesis*. It is illustrative to review some of the points made by the authors, as they have general applicability. They note that in the early 1980s, many knowledgeable people believed that cochlear implants would provide only modest awareness of ambient sounds and that speech recognition was a highly unlikely outcome. It is fair to say that the evolution in electronics from that time made the available toolkit much more complete for both compact spectral analysis chips and electrode design. Viewed as an opportunity for product development in the early 80s, even by a large company, one would have concluded without doubt that the task was impossible. Here is a case where dogged researchers and unrelated consumer and business electronics developments altered the landscape drastically by the mid-90s. This is an important point, for the intent of the current review is *not* to suggest that some lines of research should be abandoned (e.g., the silicon retina), only that translational goals must be near-term (years, not decades) for any sensible advancements in actual patient-worthy device development. Though cardiac pacing had been around for some time when cochlear implants became a serious possibility, the field of neuromodulation was relatively new and one may appropriately classify cochlear implants as neuromodulators. One other lesson to emphasize from Wilson et al. is that there may be unexpected resistance to adoption of a new implant technology. In the case of the cochlear implant, it was the deaf community itself. Though by no means universal, there was nonetheless some pushback on the idea that deaf children (for whom the success with early intervention is the greatest) must regain hearing to be productive people and citizens. The historical struggle of deaf people to gain respect and proper recognition could understandably lead to a perception that cochlear implants were meant as salvations of some sort, even if this was not at all in the minds of the developers of the technology. Today, there is a generally balanced view that cochlear implant recipients should not be stigmatized, one way or the other and that, at best, the implants are still tools to assist the user, not unlike the corrective action of glasses or hearing aids.

8.3 CURRENT TRENDS IN FDA REGULATIONS

A presentation by Dr. William Maisel, Deputy Center Director for Science and Chief Scientist, Center for Devices and Radiological Health (CDRH) at MEDCON 2011 provides insight into areas where the FDA expects growth (CDRH is the branch of the FDA that regulates medical devices). His list of emerging trends includes several areas wherein sensors, either alone or in a system, will be relevant:

- Robotics
- Miniaturized devices (nanotechnology)
- Combination products
- Sophisticated, computer-related technologies
- Organ replacements and assist devices
- Personalized medicine
- Wireless systems
- Home use

He also defined the CDRH Innovation Initiative:

- Facilitate the development and regulatory evaluation of innovative medical devices
- Strengthen the U.S. research infrastructure and promote high-quality regulatory science
- Prepare for and respond to transformative innovative technologies and scientific breakthroughs

This summary parallels a report [28] by CDRH in which fifteen non-FDA medical device experts were polled about technology developments in the device field. In particular the committee highlighted photonic and acoustic devices as being "invasiveness-reducing" and sensor technologies in general for detection, diagnosis, and monitoring.

One of the frequent mistakes made by companies during the development of new devices is to avoid talking to the FDA early in the process. This does not mean calling the FDA to ask frequent, minor questions, but it is important to talk about strategy before going too far down the development path. For example, a primary determination for devices is whether they present a significant or non-significant risk to the patient (SR or NSR). If a device is found to be SR, then its use in patients must wait until an investigational device exemption (IDE) is approved. If however an IRB (Institutional Review Board) agrees that a device is NSR, then clinical studies can proceed under IRB approval only. Most implanted sensor devices will be considered SR and therefore an IDE approval must precede clinical use.

The new guidelines on the *de novo* regulatory structure will have a significant potential impact on implanted devices. As explained earlier, this category is meant to deal with devices that do not have obvious predicates (substantial equivalence), but nonetheless are not Class III devices (presenting a major risk to health and well-being of the patient). The ability to claim substantial equivalence for novel devices

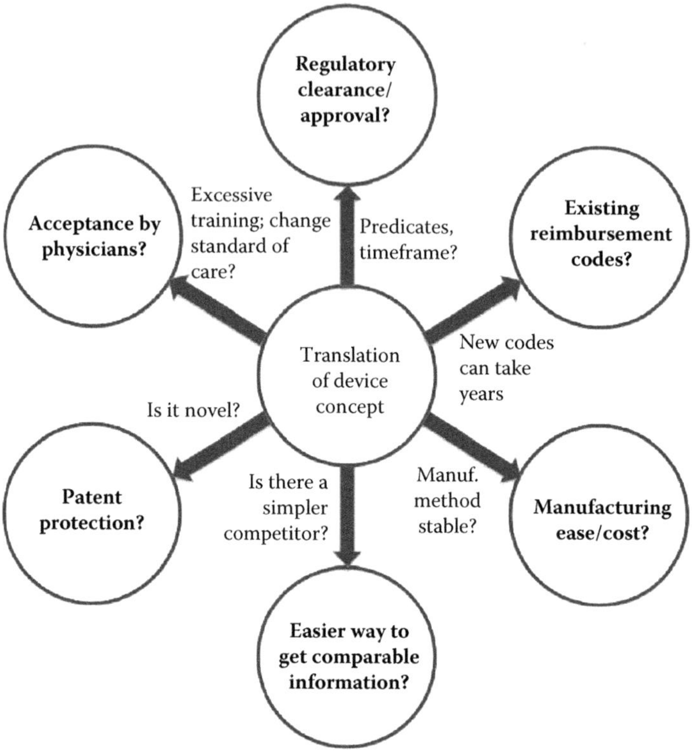

FIGURE 8.2 The interplay of essential questions that should be addressed even in the earliest stages of medical device/sensor development.

has become more limited in the last several years, especially in the use of combination predicates (using two or more separate existing devices to match to the new product). Without a strong *de novo* mechanism, therefore, devices that should rightly have Class II designation are forced into a PMA approval path. Though the *de novo* system has been around for a number of years, it has been used very infrequently, mostly because of residual confusion as to when it should be applied and a degree of uneven responsiveness within the FDA. This has led to a significant movement of early device sales outside the United States, where often devices that would be Class II in the United States are granted market clearance (e.g., via the CE mark). The U.S. medical device community is looking hopefully at a re-energized *de novo* process to provide more tractable early access to U.S. patients.

8.4 SUMMARY

The concept of personalized medicine has not come to pass as rapidly as expected based on the number of encouraging, perhaps overly naïve, press releases describing new patient-specific devices, often based on advanced sensor technology. However, drawing from the lesson of cochlear implants, there are several factors that come to bear: the maturity of the technical approach, the translatability to the clinic, and the degree to which physicians and patients accept new technology. Several decades of work and refinement were needed before cochlear implants became practical. By comparison, the Pill Cam was adopted fairly rapidly since the technology, small imaging arrays and transmitters, had undergone significant refinement in the commercial electronics sector. Additionally, minimally invasive imaging of the small intestine was an application in search of a solution and thus physician acceptance was rapid. Finally, the story of continuous glucose monitoring is illustrative in that the "ultimate" sensor system, one that would be fully implantable, proved to be too challenging and an intermediate approach, limited-duration percutaneous sensor implants, allowed manufacturers, patients, and physicians to provide greater control and convenience sooner. Sensor researchers who wish to impact medicine need to think expansively and consider the trajectory of their work beyond the laboratory/discovery phase. It is important to not only manage the expectations of future patients, but their own predictions and motivations as they embark on what can be vital and fulfilling work.

REFERENCES

1. J.H.M. Bergmann, V. Chandaria, et al. "Wearable and implantable sensors: The patient's perspective." *Sensors* 12: 16695–16709, 2012.
2. R.D. Black. "Recent advances in translational work on implantable sensors." *IEEE Sensors Journal* 11(12): 3171–3182, 2011.
3. E.H. Ledet, D. D'Lima, et al. "Implantable sensor technology: from research to clinical practice." *J Am Acad Orthop Surg* 20(6): 383–392, 2012.
4. A. Inmann and Hodgins, D., eds. *Implantable Sensor Systems for Medical Applications*, vol. 52, Philadelphia, PA: Woodhead, 2013.
5. J.J. Smith and J.A. Henderson. FDA Regulation of Implantable Sensors: Demonstrating Safety and Effectiveness for Marketing in the U.S." *IEEE Sensors Journal* 8(1): 52–56, 2008.
6. W.V. Tamborlane, et al. "Continuous glucose monitoring and intensive treatment of type 1 diabetes," *N Engl J Med* 359:1464–1476, Oct. 2, 2008.
7. D. Raccah, et al. "Incremental value of continuous glucose monitoring when starting pump therapy in patients with poorly controlled type 1 diabetes: The RealTrend study," *Diabetes Care* 32:2245–2250, Dec. 2009.
8. I. Conget, et al. "The SWITCH study (sensing with insulin pump therapy to control HbA(1c)): Design and methods of a randomized controlled crossover trial on sensor-augmented insulin pump efficacy in type 1 diabetes suboptimally controlled with pump therapy," *Diabetes Technol Ther* 13:49–54, Jan. 2011.
9. K. Nishida, et al. "What is artificial endocrine pancreas? Mechanism and history," *World J Gastroenterol* 15: 4105–4110, Sep. 7 2009.
10. R.R. Rubin, et al. "Crossing the technology divide: Practical strategies for transitioning patients from multiple daily insulin injections to sensor-augmented pump therapy," *Diabetes Educ* 37(1):5S-18S; quiz 19S-20S, Jan.–Feb. 2011.
11. J. Hermanides, et al. "Sensor-augmented insulin pump therapy to treat hyperglycemia at the coronary care unit: A randomized clinical pilot trial," *Diabetes Technol Ther* 12:537–542, Jul. 2010.
12. T. Klupa, et al. "Use of sensor-augmented insulin pump in patient with diabetes and cystic fibrosis: Evidence for improvement in metabolic control, " *Diabetes Technol Ther* 10:46–49, Feb. 2008.

13. J.R. Castle and W.K. Ward. "Amperometric glucose sensors: Sources of error and potential benefit of redundancy, " *J Diabetes Sci Technol* 4:221–225, Jan. 2010.
14. H. Takaoka and M. Yasuzawa. "Fabrication of an implantable fine needle-type glucose sensor using gamma-polyglutamic acid," *Anal Sci* 26:551–555, 2010.
15. J.N. Patel, et al. "Flexible glucose sensor utilizing multilayer PDMS process," *Conf Proc IEEE Eng Med Biol Soc* 2008:5749–5752, 2008.
16. L. Qiang, et al. "Edge-plane microwire electrodes for highly sensitive H(2)O(2) and glucose detection," *Biosens Bioelectron* 26:3755–3760, Feb. 18, 2011.
17. O. Yehezkeli, et al. "Integrated oligoaniline-cross-linked composites of Au nanoparticles/glucose oxidase electrodes: A generic paradigm for electrically contacted enzyme systems," *Chemistry* 15: 2674–2679, Mar. 2, 2009.
18. D.A. Gough, et al. "Function of an implanted tissue glucose sensor for more than 1 year in animals," *Sci Transl Med* 2:42–53, Jul. 28, 2010.
19. E.W. Stein, et al. "Microscale enzymatic optical biosensors using mass transport limiting nanofilms. 2. Response modulation by varying analyte transport properties," *Anal Chem* 80:1408–1417, Mar. 1, 2008.
20. R. Long and M. McShane. "Three-dimensional, multiwavelength Monte Carlo simulations of dermally implantable luminescent sensors," *J Biomed Opt* 15(2):027011-1–07711-13, Mar.–Apr. 2010.
21. S. Singh and M. McShane. "Enhancing the longevity of microparticle-based glucose sensors towards 1 month continuous operation," *Biosens Bioelectron* 25:1075–1081, Jan. 15, 2010.
22. S. Singh and M. McShane. "Role of porosity in tuning the response range of microsphere-based glucose sensors," *Biosens Bioelectron* 26:2478–2483, Jan. 15, 2011.
23. A. Chaudhary, et al. "Glucose response of dissolved-core alginate microspheres: Towards a continuous glucose biosensor," *Analyst* 135:2620–2628, Oct. 2010.
24. R.D. Jayant, et al. "*In vitro* and *in vivo* evaluation of anti-inflammatory agents using nanoengineered alginate carriers: Towards localized implant inflammation suppression," *Int J Pharm* 403:268–275, Jan. 17, 2011.
25. P. Valdastri, et al. "Wireless implantable electronic platform for chronic fluorescent-based biosensors," *IEEE Trans Biomed Eng* 58:1846–1854, Jun. 2011.
26. J.V. Veetil, et al. "A glucose sensor protein for continuous glucose monitoring," *Biosens Bioelectron* 26:1650–1655, Dec. 15 2010.
27. Wilson, B.S. and M.F. Dorman. "Interfacing sensors with the nervous system: Lessons from the development and success of the cochlear implant," *IEEE Sensors Journal* 8:131–147, 2008.
28. Future Trends in Medical Device Technologies: A Ten-Year Forecast (www.fda.gov/downloads/AboutFDA/CentersOffices/CDRH/CDRHReports/UCM238527.pdf). Accessed 4/7/14.

Index

C

D

K

L

M

N

O

P

Q

R

S

V

W

For Product Safety Concerns and Information please contact our EU representative GPSR@taylorandfrancis.com Taylor & Francis Verlag GmbH, Kaufingerstraße 24, 80331 München, Germany

Batch number: 10725802

Printed by Printforce, the Netherlands